AMERICAN
IDLE

ALSO BY MARY COLLINS

The Essential Daughter: Changing Expectations for Girls at Home (Praeger)
National Public Radio (Seven Locks Press)
Airborne: A Photobiography of Wilbur and Orville Wright (National Geographic Books)

OTHER TITLES IN THE CAPITAL IDEAS SERIES

*BABY AT RISK: The Uncertain Legacies of
Medical Miracles for Babies, Families, and Society*
—by Ruth Levy Guyer

DAYDREAMS AT WORK: Wake Up Your Creative Powers
—by Amy Fries

*DIGITALLY DAUNTED: The Consumer's Guide to Taking Control of
the Technology in Your Life*
—by Sean Westcott and Jean Riescher Westcott

HITTING YOUR STRIDE: Your Work, Your Way
—by Nan S. Russell

LIKE, WHATEVER: The Insider's Guide to Raising Teens
—edited by Rebecca Kahlenberg

*MARCH TO A PROMISED LAND: The Civil Rights Files of a
White Reporter (1952-1968)*
—by Al Kuettner

PROTECT YOURSELF AT COLLEGE: Smart Choices—Safe Results
—by Thomas M. Kane

DO THE RIGHT THING: PR Tips for a Skeptical Public
—by James Hoggan with Richard Littlemore

SAVE THE WORLD AND STILL BE HOME FOR DINNER
—by Will Marré

VOCABULARY OF SUCCESS: 403 Words Smart People Should Know
—by C. Edward Good

AMERICAN

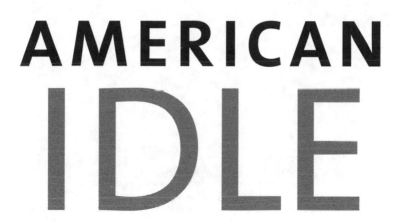

IDLE

A Journey Through Our Sedentary Culture

Mary Collins

Capital Ideas Series

CAPITAL
BOOKS, INC.
Sterling, Virginia

Capital Books, Inc.
P.O. Box 605
Herndon, Virginia 20172-0605

ISBN 13: 978-1-933102-88-7

Library of Congress Cataloging-in-Publication Data
Collins, Mary, 1961-
   American idle : a journey through our sedentary culture / Mary Collins. — 1st ed.
      p. ; cm.— (Capital ideas series)
   Includes bibliographical references.
   ISBN-13: 978-1-933102-88-7 (alk. paper)
   ISBN-10: 1-933102-88-8 (alk. paper)
   1. Exercise—United States. 2. Health behavior—United States. 3. Physical fitness—United States. I. Title. II. Series: Capital ideas series.
   [DNLM: 1. Motor Activity—United States. 2. Health Behavior—United States. 3. Health Policy—United States. 4. Life Style—United States. 5. Physical Fitness—United States. WE 103 C712a 2009]

   QP301.C5865 2009
   612.7'6—dc22

                                        2009014994

Printed in the United States of America on acid-free paper that meets the American National Standards Institute Z39-48 Standard.

First Edition

10 9 8 7 6 5 4 3 2 1

Photograph used in chapter headings by Etienne-Jules Marey. For more images by this groundbreaking nineteenth-century photographer and expert in human motion, visit Mary Collins' website, marycollinswriter.net.

To Tricia
my sister and best friend
with love

Contents

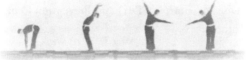

Foreword

In 2000, Mary Collins got into a bicycle crash in Alexandria, Virginia, a densely populated suburb outside of Washington, D.C. She suffered multiple crushing injuries; some that would be repaired over time, and some that she would have to learn to live with, including ruptured disks in her back and a damaged sense of hearing and smell. I have only known Mary in her post-crash life. I came to know her because she was writing this book, and I was one of the many cold calls she made as part of her research. Mary describes our meeting in one of her chapters so I won't do it here. What I will do is tell you that despite a loss of hearing, Mary is a gifted listener and an extraordinary storyteller. This book is part travel, part autobiographical, part research. It's an artichoke—part vegetable, part flower, many interesting layers. Urban planners, anthropologists, archeologists, public-health professionals, sports trainers, historians, scientists, adventurers, and just about anyone who has an interest in people and places will find something to connect to in *American Idle*.

I believe Mary wrote the book because she experienced the loss of her physical self—a self that she had been very proud of as an athlete. Her physical comeback has been hard fought, and it caused her to look at human behavior and modern lifestyle trends in a different way and with a deeper sensitivity, in the same way we might appreciate the absence of pain only when we are in pain or appreciate walking only when we are immobilized. Without realizing it, many of us have lapsed into a state of being idle, and unlike the bear that Mary describes in her visit to the National Zoo, "We cannot convert nitrogen into protein, go months without drinking or urinating, or retain bone mass without moving." A bear can emerge from its cave at the end of winter and move right into bear society without an intense regimen of physical therapy or pharmaceuticals. Figuratively speaking, a bear could go from cave to bicycle and do it well. Humans, on the other hand, are a different story.

Movement is essential to our well-being. The cessation of movement or the gradual withdrawal from everyday activity is why more than 20 percent of adults are obese in every state except Colorado and why children are increasingly being diagnosed with heart disease and diabetes. Too many of us are ignoring the basic truth about our own health and well-being and have fallen asleep in the poppy fields drunk with the machines that let us remain idle. Too many of us, for example, view March as a time to watch the Final Four from the comforts of a soft couch or a seat at the bar, rather than a great time to enjoy a bicycle ride, a brisk run, or a walk around the neighborhood to go crocus spotting, mail a letter, or string a few errands together.

Forty percent of all trips made in the United States are just two miles or less and yet the vast majority of all trips are made by car. These short trips are the easiest to shift to bicycling and walking and also the most polluting and energy intensive. But rarely do we consider the benefits of walking and bicycling, the costs of not walking or bicycling, or the cumulative impact of not being physically active. Rarely do we consider the public policies that make it difficult to walk or bike, favor highways over walkways, and that promote big-box land use. Too many parents are afraid to let their children go out and play, and we've become okay with that. In a single generation, we have gone from a nation where most kids walk or bike to school to one where fewer than 15 percent do. If the trend continues, the walk to school will begin to sound like a Paul Bunyan tale.

As the executive director of the National Center for Bicycling & Walking, promoting walking and bicycling is a full-time job for me. I promote these activities not only because of the physical benefits, but also because if we replaced even some of the trips we make by automobiles with bicycling or walking, the polar bear cubs wouldn't be drowning and, closer to home, not as many kids would be suffering from respiratory diseases. If we invested in making roadways and communities safer for bicyclists and pedestrians, it is likely that more people, including children, would walk and bike; and most importantly, they would arrive alive, and as some studies point out, more intellectually stimulated.

Nationally, pedestrians and bicyclists account for 13 percent of roadway fatalities, but less than 1 percent of safety funding is spent on improvements to make roads safer for pedestrians and bicyclists. Removing the barriers to walking and biking and making these activities safer, convenient, and more viable will go a long way to getting people out of their caves and on their heels.

I don't know the details of the crash that nearly paralyzed Mary; her loss of memory of that incident makes it impossible to retell the story. But it is quite possible that if we invested a little more into safe and complete streets—the kinds of streets that accommodate motor vehicles as well as bicycles and pedestrians—Mary would not have been run over. Walking and biking are like frogs—the indicator species of a healthy place. These activities bring us to places where we interact more with people and the environment.

This book will introduce you to people like Jane Jacobs, author of *The Death and Life of Great American Cities*, and a champion for social and environmental justice long before those phrases had a defined meaning. Ms. Jacobs understood the importance of preserving places people could move through on foot; *American Idle* continues and expands on Jacobs' line of thought.

In elementary school, we learn about the settling of the West, the great expedition of Lewis and Clark, the marchers in the Civil Rights movement; but few of us ever stop to think about the vital role of physical movement in these great American moments. Under the power of Mary's pen, we are reminded of this and of the current skewed ratio of stillness to movement in our daily lives. By interviewing a huge range of people, Mary captures the habits and thoughts of the young, the old, the immigrant, and the expert.

I recently picked up a copy of John Steinbeck's *Cannery Row*. In the introduction, Steinbeck writes about collecting marine animals. He describes ". . . certain flat worms as being so delicate that they are almost impossible to capture whole. You must let them ooze and crawl of their own will onto a knife blade and then lift gently into your bottle of sea water. And perhaps that might be the best way to read this book—to open the page and to let the stories crawl in by themselves."

When I read that last line, I thought of this book. The best way to read *American Idle* is to let the stories—Mary's story, the story of our cultural and physical de-evolution into a sedentary state, and the stories of all the people she interviewed—crawl in.

But understand there is a cautionary tale here. As human beings, our future, our ability to remain vibrant healthy beings, depends on a steady diet of activity. We can be boards or we can be sponges. Boards are stiff and rigid. They stay in place. Sponges absorb and flex; with a little water they spring into action.

—SHARON Z. ROERTY
EXECUTIVE DIRECTOR, NATIONAL CENTER FOR
BICYCLING & WALKING

Acknowledgments

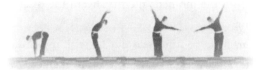

Writing is always a group activity, especially when you stand alone in front of the screen and type. I never would have stuck with this project if I hadn't always felt the presence of my attentive outside readers waiting for my next chapter, in particular my mother, Constance Collins Cain; my sister, Betty Collins; and my colleague and friend, Susan Tejada. My brother, Jim Collins, gave me indispensable advice as I negotiated talks with editors at various publishing houses. I must also add a special line for my agent, Kathi Paton, who took on a literary nonfiction manuscript in a hard market and never gave up on it. She offered outstanding editorial advice and even came up with the book's witty title.

While researching the book, dozens of people gave generously of their time and expertise: Sharon Roerty, of the National Center for Bicycling & Walking; Bill Sands, at the United States Olympic Center; Karen Bradley, of the Laban/Bertenieff Institute of Movement; Dr. Fred Gage, of the Salk Institute; Dr. Thomas Farley, of Tulane University; Kevin Coyle, of the National Wildlife Federation; Dr. Steve Holden, from the Denver Museum of Nature and Science; Dr. Rolfe Mandel, of the University of Kansas; Keith Laughlin, of Rails and Trails; Matilde Palmer; Rachel Winch; Harrison Taylor Godfrey; John Gibbons; and many other individuals whom I interviewed.

I wish to thank Central Connecticut State University and the AAUP chapter at CCSU for providing crucial financial support so I could complete the final revisions of this book. And even though I am no longer teaching at Johns Hopkins University's Master of Arts in Writing program in Washington, D.C.,

I must thank all of the splendid students and colleagues I knew while working there and who kept me motivated during the crucial first two years on this project.

Amy Fries at Capital Books is an outstanding editor and championed my project right from the moment she first heard me discuss my manuscript at a Hopkins' event.

My daughter, Julia, continues to put up with my endless tapping at the keyboard as I write and write and write. I want to thank her for adding such a wonderful blend of humor, beauty, and light to my life.

Introduction

Reclaiming Our Physical Selves

I have no memory of the bicycle accident that inspired this book or the helicopter ride that swooped me to the Washington Hospital Trauma Center in the nation's capital. The people who found me and called 911 thought I had broken my neck.

I did eventually need back surgery to repair some ruptured disks, but I regained full feeling and full motion. What I lost: my life as a former varsity college athlete, avid basketball player, and runner. What I found: a whole new way of thinking about my body, about the role of movement in my life and all of our lives. With one ill-fated slip of my bicycle wheel, I became more like the average American. I began to count myself lucky if I engaged in moderate exercise three times a week.

The shift wasn't just difficult for me; it was absolutely life altering on every level and impacted my social life, my moods, my ability to work and focus. I decided as I rebuilt my body I would also embark on a journey to see what could be done about the broken national body. I had read again and again that 65 percent of Americans are overweight or obese and engage in moderate activity less than three times a week. Record numbers of us suffer from heart disease, diabetes, and a host of other lifestyle-related problems. For the first time, the younger generation may live shorter, less vital lives than their parents, despite advances in medical care. Essentially, our culture has immobilized us as effectively as a shattered body part.

After years of hard work, I no longer live like a wounded bird, but most Americans do. This book asks why and explores the forces that put us in that mindset and the forces we need to harness to push it away. I trace the lost movement in our lives and the physical, social, cultural, and even moral consequences of that loss.

I have always loved history and archeology, so when I read about a dig in Kanorado, Kansas, that showed evidence of humans who may have trekked to the heartland as long as 14,000 years ago, I knew where I needed to start my *American Idle* project. For most of human history people have lived as hunter-gatherers, which means our bodies evolved over hundreds of thousands of years to meet the demands of that lifestyle. What did it mean that for 99 percent of human history we lived as a species on the move?

Today, of course, we read words, but forgot how to read landscapes by walking through them. We turn pages with our index finger, but no longer know what it feels like to constantly use our hands to simply survive. We have stopped ourselves in our tracks. Each week we might *choose* to exercise for the sake of fitness, weight loss, or pleasure, but most of us no longer have to.

I have no desire to idealize the past. Our ancient ancestors died young, usually before age fifty, and lived hard with no answer for arthritis or joints worn out from overuse. But their hard times and our soft ones do not change our mutual physical legacy: we are meant to move—often—at all sorts of speeds and over all sorts of terrain.

As I learned when I went to the dig in Kanorado, there was no one standard hunter-gatherer pattern of life—some groups fished, others hunted big game—but all shared the common need to move to stay alive. Any portrait of our distant past would be incomplete without the image of the upright, long-distance trekker.

I held tools crafted and carried on foot by one of these trekkers as I stood in the Kansas summer sun. Sweat collected in all the bends in my body; cars and trucks whizzed by on the overpass above me. I can't even imagine walking these huge, flat plains for weeks on end, following the water and game; but the sensation of standing there in the open palm of the land made me glad I had decided to go on location to see things for myself. In that moment, I knew I had to continue to build up my strength so I could travel to all sorts of locations to complete my story about our physical legacy. For someone who couldn't last more than a few hours in a chair, this was a major objective, which proved incredibly motivating as I tried to stick with my swimming, walking, and physical-therapy routine.

Of course, I also visited books and scholarly journals and learned that I didn't have to dig in the dirt to uncover our physical past; I could simply look at my own body, which has more sweat glands than nearly any other animal and as many fat cells as a polar bear. Once trained, humans are able to move over long distances, replenish themselves with water and food, and relieve themselves of heat under a hot sun better than nearly any other creature that's ever lived on Earth. We're long trekkers right down to the shape of our ankle.

And yet here we sit.

As I tried to cope with the balance of movement and stillness in my own life, I learned how other species handle that all-important ratio. I eventually went to the National Zoo in Washington, D.C., and walked the grounds with John Gibbons, a zoo employee, who helped me get a better feel for where we fall on the movement continuum on Earth. I learned that the peregrine falcon is the first place winner in the speed category, since it can dive 200 miles per hour as it strikes prey, and that creatures like the three-toed sloth use stillness as a clever survival tool. Ancient humans fall on the upper range of the activity pyramid of mammals, though near the bottom third if you include insects and fish.

Modern humans, well, it's a little unclear, since we expend only about a third of the physical energy our ancient ancestors burned, but the answer to the question has clearly changed. As Gibbons pointed out during my visit with him, movement and food are intricately linked. If we can feed ourselves by simply walking into the kitchen for a snack, we'll do that and won't feel pressured to do more. Most captive animals slip into the same trap, which means they often suffer from obesity, nervous disorders, depression, and other health problems too.

Animals at the zoo remain still most of the time. Of course living in an enclosure limits movement, but even in the wild, nature makes ample use of rest. A cheetah may be able to reach speeds of 60 miles per hour, but it spends at least fifteen hours of every day asleep. The silverback lowland gorilla has cords of muscles under his chest, but he hangs in his nest a large part of every day. For many creatures stillness is a way of life—a trick that they often couple with camouflage. They live longer if they do less.

For many Americans, that seems the perfect equation, which partially accounts for scientists' interest in bears, which gorge for weeks in late summer and then hibernate for months in winter. In early spring they emerge thinner and at full strength. A human who laid down for half as long would be like an astronaut coming home from a gravity-free environment—weak-kneed and suffering from bone loss. Unlike the bear, we cannot convert nitrogen into protein, go months without drinking or urinating, or retain bone mass without moving. Some scientists hope to unlock some of the bears' secrets and transfer them to humans; but nature has a carefully calibrated movement contract with each species, and a quick fix "bear pill" may prove a dangerous illusion. Our best bet: embrace our own legacy.

So how did we get so dislocated from that legacy? Well, farming and then the Industrial Revolution hit our species and shattered our unbroken history as long-distance movers. Essentially these events were the bicycle accident of our past.

Today a farm actually stands on the prehistoric artifacts in Kanorado, which is another reason why this speck of a town proved a perfect starting point for a quest to retrace our physical story. Black steer sniff out pools of water near a cut in the soil that holds mammoth bones and ancient hide scrapers. Until 1920, more than half of Americans still lived on farms, harrowing their fields and hauling water from wells. Today, less than 5 percent do, and most of them work their land with enormous machines, like the ones I spied near the silos on my drive to the site; most contemporary farmers burn gasoline, not calories.

The shift to office work began well before 1920, however, and with it the growing divide between physical activity and labor. By the 1850s, authors—like Cate Beecher, sister of Harriet Beecher Stowe of *Uncle Tom's Cabin* fame—wrote bestsellers about the health problems caused by a gradual shift from farm life to city life and desk jobs, including depression, back problems, and anxiety disorders.

In *Letters to the People on Health and Happiness,* Beecher tapped into a deep vein of panic among Americans in the nineteenth century, who began to wonder how a generation of men working desk jobs could ever muster the physical strength to defend a nation in a time of war. Scientists—like Dr. Dudley Allen Sargent of Harvard University, who invented fitness equipment that served as a forerunner to machines such as the StairMaster—began to push for much more rigorous leisure activities. Bicycle riding took off by the late 1800s, and for the first time members of both sexes and all ages could go out for long recreational rides and enter competitive races that required training. The Pope Manufacturing Company, the biggest producer of bicycles in the U.S., was based in my hometown of Hartford, Connecticut, which made it the center for both Beechers, who lived there, and the new recreational fad. By 1900 almost half of Americans had lives clearly divided between their work and their physical activity. Movement had become something separate from the rest of their day.

Colleges added organized sports at record rates. Public schools began requiring physical education classes. And still, the average American's overall fitness level declined. Thanks to advances in modern medicine, life expectancy went up, but the amount the average adult moved each day dropped off dramatically.

By the opening of the twentieth century, the crisis had only deepened, especially in the workplace, as manufacturers became increasingly focused on cost-effective, efficient assembly lines. Time-management experts, such as Frederick Winslow Taylor, developed systems that made each action a careful piece of a chain of actions centered on speed and productivity. At places like the Ford Motor Company, a man might perform the same task nine to ten hours a day, five to six days a week. The turnover rate in some jobs reached 900 percent a year.

To fully understand movement as a means of production, I left the Beechers and bicycles and headed to factories in Pennsylvania. There I watched blue-aproned women scan for burnt potato chips as a conveyor belt moved 3,000 chips past them in an hour, and gagged on the oil-thick air of a Harley Davidson motorcycle plant, where workers turn out 850 bikes a day on a line that moves six feet a minute. There's no grace on these table-flat factory floors, just repetitive motion injuries and workers oddly on the move and yet immobile at the same time. At the Utz Potato Chip factory all of the workers knew the occupational nurse.

Clearly something about the jobs on the factory floor was not right for the workers' bodies, but how should we define "right" for the modern physical human? I went to the U.S. Olympic Center (USOC) in Colorado Springs, Colorado, in search of the ultimate physical success story. Surely our combination of know-how and training was producing some of the finest physical specimens ever known to man.

But as my conversations with Bill Sands, director of Sports Science at the USOC, soon made clear, while the modern professional athlete is a remarkable specimen, the much bigger and more relevant story is the growing physical divide between the elite pro and the average Joe.

The entire sports culture, right down to the youth-league level, has made fitness—and the physical grace and body awareness that accompanies it—something that children and adults usually acquire only in supervised, and often competitive, programs. The spontaneous physical flow that characterized life for our hunter-gatherer ancestors on the Great Plains has been lost. Even the ultimate sports director of the ultimate sports team believes this is a devastating shift that impacts not only the physical, but also the spiritual center of our society.

"With the exception of athletes, dancers, and soldiers, everyone else has lost physical grace," he said.

By the time I left the USOC facility I knew my trip through America's physical past and present had taken on many more layers of meaning. I was no longer just looking for the athlete's vision of a fit life, but something more nuanced and all-encompassing, something that celebrated incorporating all forms of movement in as many different peoples' lives as possible and in ways that had nothing to do with medals and record times.

Once again, after a physical trip to a place, I returned home to research my next step, which, after Colorado, actually brought me online to the federal government websites to see what's being done at the highest levels to close the Olympian gap between trained athletes and the typical citizen.

The government has advocated a minimum of thirty minutes of activity five days a week since the *Eisenhower* administration. At the time, 65 percent of Americans failed to meet this modest objective. Even more baffling, after decades of advertising, wellness initiatives, headlines in national news outlets, and billions of dollars, that percentage has remained unchanged.

Clearly getting the word out and sponsoring a wellness day here and there is not working. I pressed onward in my web journey and came across a "Barriers to Being Active Quiz" on the Centers for Disease Control and Prevention (CDC) webpage that cuts closer to the root of our collective inertia. A summary of quiz results showed that Americans neglect their physical fitness for three primary reasons: lack of time, lack of access to trails and parks, and fear of strangers in public places.

My man-in-the-street interviews across the country confirm the CDC results. As one young, white, professional woman in Washington, D.C., told me: "Even those of us for whom all of this is central to our lives, who care deeply about physical activity and nutrition, the conditions are stacked against us."

So personal responsibility only goes so far; lots of things out there that we feel we can't control contribute to our biblical levels of slothfulness. Studies show that something as simple as a bike path near a neighborhood can increase people's activity levels as much as 25 percent.

But *fear* and *lack* are hard to get a handle on, slippery abstractions that require not just physical changes in the landscape but *emotional* and *mental* changes in individuals. I traveled to a conference in San Diego, California, which pulled together urban planners, wellness directors, sociologists, and public-health experts interested in precisely these more abstract issues that lie at the root of Americans' declining physical-activity levels.

Sponsored by the Active Living Research Foundation, a nonprofit group that played a major role in successful anti-smoking campaigns, the conference ran over two days and covered everything from bringing light rail and sidewalks to cities to organizing campaigns to encourage kids to walk or bike to school.

In his keynote address, Dr. Thomas Farley, professor of public health at Tulane University in New Orleans and author of *A Prescription for a Healthy Nation,* claimed that the hurricane-ravaged area in Louisiana could serve as a blank slate for a whole new approach to city planning that would make diet and physical activity central to design. He talked of light rail, more public parks, and a special tax break for grocers who sold vegetables and fresh fruit instead of soda and chips. In his book, he makes clear that *preventive* medicine—clean water, better diet, better sewage disposal, and exercise—and not surgery or even vaccines, has accounted for 85 percent of the rise in life expectancy since 1890. And what better place to try out new preventive measures than in a state that ranks forty-ninth in adult and infant mortality?

But even as he shared the dream with a very receptive audience, Farley conceded that most of these ideas have not been included in the rebuilding plans to date. At one point when he attended a neighborhood association meeting, the residents wanted to hear about filling potholes or securing a stop sign. It never crossed anyone's mind to discuss something as abstract as a snack-food tax or as ambitious as light rail.

I later learned that Farley, and other members of the faculty at Tulane University, had teamed up with the CDC in 2007 to create Partnership for an Active Community Environment (PACE), which will introduce many of the ideas that Farley discussed into one sample neighborhood—the Upper Ninth Ward—as part of a five-year experiment. They will look at how more parks, walkways, better lighting, better access to good food, etc., can alter the physical activity and dietary habits of even the most at-risk poor populations.

At the time, Farley did not mention PACE, and I walked away from his talk discouraged. It took generations to get us where we are and it may take generations to get us back to a more balanced place. In the meantime, the social, physical, and even spiritual costs keep mounting.

Feeling moody and nursing a beer, I sat at a bar by myself.

But then Sharon Roerty, executive director of the National Center for Bicycling & Walking and fellow conference attendee, pulled up a seat. She goes into cities like Baltimore and spreads the gospel of "getting movement into the flow of everyday life," as she describes it. She shows anyone who will listen how safe public spaces build close community connections, how kids who walk or bike to school concentrate better and have fewer behavioral problems. She makes it clear that weight loss and toned muscles are not the greatest benefits of a more physical daily life.

In no time the Jersey native brought me over to her more hopeful, proactive way of thinking. We agreed to tackle New York City together on foot so we could see firsthand how and why it works as one of America's most walkable urban spaces.

A month after the conference, I trekked 25,000 steps through the Lower East Side, Soho, Chinatown, and Central Park in Manhattan with Sharon as my guide. As we moved along the crowded sidewalks, we discussed the history of urban planning in the United States, especially the work of community advocate Jane Jacobs, who saved neighborhoods in New York City from the wrecking ball in the 1960s when she helped defeat an Expressway slated to run through Soho.

In *The Death and Life of Great American Cities*, Jacobs wrote about the importance of living in a world built on a human scale. Her book became a bible of sorts for the contemporary Smart Growth movement, but it's not just a paean to intelligent urban planning. Many of her best ideas centered on ways to keep people moving on foot through public spaces. A neighborhood built to scale is also a neighborhood designed for daily spontaneous exercise.

By the time I reached Sheep's Meadow in Central Park with Sharon, I had traveled back and forth across the United States by car, airplane, and on foot, and I knew I had finally found someone with the vision we all need. Sharon, more than anyone I spoke with, fully understands that the way we physically move through our days profoundly impacts our physical, social, even spiritual well-being.

This is what Americans need to hear. This is the far more nuanced story that the federal government and nonprofit groups, like the American Heart Association, need to tell. Our sedentary culture not only eats away at our bodies but also our community lives, our spiritual center, and the fundamental threads of a healthy society. How could 65 percent of Americans hear that more complex story—I mean truly *hear*—and remain in their chairs?

When I returned from New York, I decided to look at the two most immobile populations in America: Hispanics and African Americans. Their collective statistics when it comes to obesity, heart disease, diabetes, and other lifestyle-related problems just rock my mind. African Americans have cancer and diabetes at *twice* the rate of whites. A ten-year-old Hispanic child living in the United States has a *50 percent* chance of developing Type 2 diabetes. And when it comes to fear and lack—no access to safe public spaces, no time, and no cash—these two groups absolutely top the list.

But the more I read the numbing details about their dismal health and habits, the more I kept thinking back to my conversation with Bill Sands at the

Olympic Center in Colorado. He had spoken of rediscovering *physical* grace, but perhaps the best way to reach these two at-risk communities was through *spiritual* grace, since both Hispanics and African Americans have strong ties to church.

I discovered Fitness Ministries, which started in white-dominated Methodist churches in the 1980s, but have since spread to all sorts of denominations. And, sure enough, when I looked through the scientific literature, I found that church-based wellness programs have a higher success rate than recreational wellness programs because participants stay with it. They overcome fear, because they work through the safest place they know; and they overcome lack, because they've already set aside time on Sundays for worship. The exercise just becomes an extension of their regular prayers.

I visited a Catholic church with a large Latino congregation, where half of the parishioners had never done any regular exercise, but faithfully carried out a re-creation of St. Paul's 3,000-mile walk through the Holy Land. I realized that the most successful programs must meet people where they *can be* and where they *want to be*, not where we wish or expect them to be. This is especially true for highly stressed at-risk populations in low-income areas.

The spiritual side of the physical story made me curious about the moral consequences as well. Every moral equation involves good and bad choices and the fallout of those choices. When it comes to diet, exercise, smoking, and alcohol, most American's make such poor decisions their lifestyle habits account for *80 percent of the healthcare costs in this country*. So something that all of us have some control over has played a huge role in the rising insurance premiums we all complain about, and the rising percentage of small businesses who cannot afford to provide insurance to their employees. Two overweight smokers in a pool of twenty workers can raise rates so high that all must be denied coverage for an employer to survive.

But the moral consequence of our sedentary lifestyle reaches even deeper than our pockets; it also reaches into our minds. Scientists have found that the growing gap between our over-stimulated brains and under-stimulated bodies can actually impair, or even completely neutralize, our ability to make moral judgments. We see uncensored and unending amounts of violence on the screen but receive no tactile input. Over time our brains shut down our natural reactions of empathy and horror and replace them with a dampened response. Modern humans are physical creatures caught in an increasingly abstract world that's confusing our hardwiring at a *chemical* level. When a boy kills a girl with a move he saw on the wrestling channel, our sedentary culture is no longer just a fitness problem.

Grace requires a refined sense of cause and effect. A physically self-aware person understands the difference between playfully flipping a kid on her back and smacking her into a table. America's sedentary culture erodes this type of body intelligence.

At the Laban/Bartenieff Institute of Movement, founded by Rudolf Laban, father of European modern dance, students study how people flow through space. They look at things like intent—Did you mean to slap her or caress her?—and notice things like the general decline in physical civility in American society.

Karen Bradley, former chair of the institute, agrees that Americans have a body-awareness problem of staggering proportions. The lack of varied physical movement throughout the day for the average person results in a mass of individuals incapable of seeing "their own impact on the world," Bradley says. Without a more sophisticated sense of self in time and space, which physical activity helps hone, it's difficult for a person to grasp cause and effect.

Bradley herself uses rhythmic dancing in her classroom work to enhance students' body awareness and timing. She also believes that dance is inherently joyful, thus recuperative, a fundamental gift inactive Americans deny themselves on a daily basis when they plop down in front of a television. Perhaps watching a screen is not the most restive way to unwind for most individuals, but few people explore other options because the media is just handed to them, literally, in a box.

For most of human history movement was precisely about that: exploring, especially in nature. At the end of my journey, I look at how the dramatic decline in free flowing physical activity has led to an even more astonishing drop in the average American's contact with the natural world. As a young girl growing up in New England in the 1960s and 1970s, I spent an hour or more each day in the woods near my home, but most of the teens in my daughter's generation rarely go outside. The average ten-year-old in 1979 wandered *ten times* farther on his or her own than a ten-year-old today.

Many books have catalogued all of the obstacles that have kept kids indoors, including the obvious and growing allure of computers, video games, and television; but few address how the frantic pace of American life makes children ill-equipped to handle a more natural flow. When my daughter's seventh-grade class went on a camping trip, most of the kids just sat on the logs around the campsite and did not want to explore or swim. They might as well have been home in front of their computer screens. Simply bringing them into the woods is no longer enough; parents and educators must now deliberately teach children how to be *in* nature.

Dr. Fred Gage, a neuroscientist at the Salk Institute in California and expert on how physical exercise impacts the brain, explained to me that all of us lose focus and mental acuity when we sit too much. That seems logical enough, of course, but what's even more startling is that Dr. Gage and his fellow researchers recently discovered that the *only* way adults can generate new neurons is through physical exercise. Working those crossword puzzles may help you *retain* neurons, but you need to *move* if you want to stem the steady drop-off in neurons in your brain as you age.

While people like Dr. Gage transformed my understanding of myself and our physical legacy as a species, I close my book with an emotional tip-of-the-hat rather than a factual bang. At journey's end, I stand in a frigid tidal pool in Maine, the land of my ancestors on my mother's side, people who worked with their hands in lumber camps, and before that, as blacksmiths in Ireland. In the first few months after my accident and before my back surgery, I had begun to lose feeling and strength in my left leg. Fully healed, in bare feet, I experienced the snapping sensation of the Atlantic Ocean in June. I knew, as I stood there, that I had successfully transformed my relationship with my own body and come closer to understanding the lives of the more physically active Americans that came before us.

When I began, I felt like a wounded bird, but emerged not only way beyond that stunted stage, but also way beyond the equally imbalanced attitude I had as a competitive college athlete. Of course my bicycle accident forced me to scale back my intensity on a physical level; I simply can't pound my body the way I used to. But where I once grieved over the shift, now I embrace it as part of an entirely new approach to moving throughout my day as regularly as possible. I credit people like Dr. Fred Gage, Sharon Roerty, and Karen Bradley for my new *mental* and *emotional* mindset. They made me see the value of sustaining a regular flow of physical movement that has nothing to do with wins or losses or weight or heart rate and everything to do with our natural rhythm as a species and all the things we lost when we let go of that.

Before I close, I want to share just one example of how a single, simple change dramatically improved the physical flow in my days. For at least two years after my back surgery, I could not sit comfortably for more than an hour or so at a time, which made it very difficult for me to run my writing and editing business. I had read somewhere that Thomas Jefferson worked at a standup desk when he wrote the Declaration of Independence, so I googled "Thomas Jefferson AND standup desk" and came upon an Amish website (of all things!), which provided information on how to contact a middleman to order a handcrafted, made-to-order standup desk.

Mine is crafted from cherry and has brass handles on the drawers that hang like bracelets on a delicate wrist. My computer screen stands at eye level and I rest my right foot on a bar, which helps to keep the bend in my lower back at the proper angle. When I become frustrated, I pace. When I tire, I swing my hips onto a tall stool, but I never sit longer than ten minutes. I can work this way for as long as six hours a day.

The Amish told me their best clients are the military officers at the Pentagon, who say they think better when they stand or roam a room.

That's what we all need to become: four-star generals of a move movement.

As I show in my conclusion, the changes don't have to be radical, just intelligent and firm. One basic standup desk transformed my office back into a workspace. In *American Idle*, I show how similar small but fundamental shifts can bring physical movement back into the flow of our everyday lives.

This book is not about losing weight, will not provide a self-help guide on how to exercise, and will not dwell on the obvious consequences of being inactive while eating a diet high in saturated fat, salt, refined flour, and sugar. Instead you will reconnect with your own physical legacy by traveling with me to the Great Plains to retrace the walking trails of prehistoric people. You will visit factory floors and see the physical sacrifices so many people make at their jobs. You will walk neighborhoods with an eye toward rebuilding community life by getting more people on foot in public spaces. You will become aware, perhaps for the first time, of the spiritual and moral costs of our sedentary lifestyle. And if you follow my journey all the way to the end, you may find your own road back to physical grace.

1

Meet the First Walkers

The American Heartland 14,000 Years Ago

I admit I am driving a car down Route 70 in Kansas, not walking like the hunter-gatherers who passed this way before me and left skin scrapers and other faint signs of their passing in the loam in a small town called Kanorado. I want to visit the oldest prehistoric campsite ever found on the Great Plains, which has stone tools that scientists call lithics, and mammoth, camel, and bison bones. I am burning gas to do it because, well, I don't have the time, muscle endurance, or inclination to trek hundreds of miles on foot. Of course most of our ancient North American ancestors had no room for such complaints and gave every ounce of energy they had to follow herds of grazing animals and to find drinkable water. I don't want to emulate the hunter-gatherer lifestyle, which was so physically demanding that few people lived past age forty-five, but I do want to trace the remarkable story of how they used their bodies.

I pull off the highway and park on a grassy field. I can see a small team of people milling around in the distance by a cut in the dirt made near a bridge off the highway. This is farm country, complete with long, flat views of dry fields, a pungent tinge of fertilizer in the air, and a few black steers by pools of water near the dig site.

Rolfe Mandel, a geologist from the University of Kansas, who supervises this archeological find, pops out of his pickup truck to greet me. An average-sized, middle-aged man with pensive features and tan safari hat, he shakes my hand and tells me to hop in.

So once again, I'm writing a book on physical activity and I find myself in a car; this time I'm only going a few hundred yards down a small slope, but I don't say anything because I'm here to play by their rules and hear their stories and theories.

The Kanorado find is big news in archeological circles because, despite decades of careful research, scientists still do not know precisely when and how the first humans settled North America. The standard theory argues that they came over the Bering Strait after the ice sheet receded about 13,500 years ago and scurried down a narrow land corridor into the American Heartland. Others think they followed the coastline of the ice sheets in boats in both the Atlantic and Pacific and settled more than 18,000 years ago in places like Virginia. Rolfe thinks the Kanorado dig may eventually unearth artifacts that date back more than 14,000 years, which would challenge the traditional Bering Strait timetable.

"That number doesn't bother me," he says, as we bounce along in his truck.

In the end, when the first people came or what direction they came from interests me less than *how* they moved across this immense landscape once they got here. The other huge story being unearthed bit by bit in Kanorado is that nearly all of the stone tools they have found came from somewhere else: Smokey Hill jasper from Nebraska, Hartville chert from Wyoming, and Alibates from the panhandle of Texas. Rolfe's colleague, archeologist Steve Holen, has developed a theory about all of these "exotics," as they call them: the hunter-gatherers carried them here on foot while trekking as much as 250 miles (400 km) twice a year in pursuit of water and game. That breaks down to something like eight to ten miles a day, which is a tall order even for seasoned soldiers, never mind a band of fifty or so people that might have included children and the elderly.

"We haven't found a single locally made lithic here. There's too much of it to claim it was just trade. People carried it here," Rolfe says as we pull up to the first of three digs in the area.

When I meet Steve, a gray-blond Richard Dreyfuss sort of person, I can see he's the funny man to Rolfe's straight guy. He likes to joke and enters in and out of a conversation with glib stories, but his blue eyes remain serious and focused. When I ask him how he got into archeology, he says, "I was born this way." I laugh, but he doesn't, because he means it.

As a boy, Steve used a mammoth tooth as a doorstop on the family farmhouse in Nebraska. His uncle, who ran a gravel pit along the Platte River, actually hated the teeth because they clogged his equipment. He didn't care that they came from animals that had lived thousands of years ago and died out for reasons that scientists still can't completely explain. But Steve cared, and he safeguarded the tooth and the other prehistoric human artifacts, like hide scrapers, which turned up in the soil on the farm as though a separate, living world existed a few feet under them.

For his doctoral research at the University of Kansas (where Rolfe served on his dissertation committee), Steve studied the spread of prehistoric stone tools across the Great Plains and concluded that the earliest Americans could cover remarkable distances. Of course these migrators hardly lived in a throwaway society. Steve has not found and probably will not find lots of stone tools or human remains dating back 12,000 to 18,000 years ago, even if people had reached the American Heartland that far back. The fact is several billion modern humans lived before the invention of agriculture 10,000 years ago, but scientists have only found the fossilized remains of a few hundred

So Steve began looking at markings on bones, especially mammoth and bison bones, and believes he's found a spiral pattern that only humans could make as they cracked them open to get at the marrow. If he's right, then the fossils he's found show that people may have traveled around the Great Plains as long as 18,000 years ago and moved distances every season that would make your car weary.

In one clever bit of dramatic research and publicity for his theory, Steve brought Alan Alda of M*A*S*H fame to the Denver Zoo. Alda was hosting a PBS special about changing ideas on how and when prehistoric settlers came to the North American continent.

In the documentary, Steve grabs some bloody beef bones and tosses them into the lions' den. Alda and Steve watch as the lions gnaw on the ends of the bones, but fail to crack them. Next, they try the hyenas, which have even more powerful jaws, but they too fail to get to the center of the bone. Finally,

Steve has Alda place the center of a thighbone on a rock and lets him hammer it with another rock. Alda's glasses slip down to the end of his nose, and he hits his hand at one point.

"I cut myself. I'm bleeding," he says. They laugh a bit, but Steve's very, very serious.

"See," he says, "you've made a spiral fracture that's unique. Only humans can make this spiral fracture," which means the mammoth bones with the tell-tale spiral fractures that he keeps finding in Nebraska, Wyoming, and now Kanorado, Kansas, were cracked open by people. Not lions, or hyenas, or the now extinct short-faced bear, but by tool-bearing hunter-gatherers who wanted to get at the marrow.

He's not the only one reaching these remarkable conclusions about prehistoric man's migrating patterns. Scientists analyzing artifacts on the great steppes of Russia have also found evidence that early people were incredible walkers. "So it looks as though they were really moving over great distances in these plains areas," Steve says. "They followed the game. And the water, of course."

By all accounts there is no such thing as the average day for an average hunter-gatherer. Most scientists agree that prehistoric people on the North American continent moved in smalls bands of fifty to a few hundred and that these small groups often interacted with other bands to exchange mates, tools, and information. Beyond that there was tremendous variety in the hunter-gatherer lifestyle. Those that lived along the shoreline, for example, didn't have to work as hard to sustain themselves as those that lived in more arid environments. But whether or not a man collected fish or a woman foraged for tubers, these people moved, sometimes as long as seven to nine hours a day. They always had to respect the unforgiving equation of food secured versus calories expended to find it.

It doesn't make much sense to travel ten miles for fruit if that fruit won't allow you to recover your calorie loss. In the few remaining hunter-gatherer cultures around the globe, the ideal circle seems to be about 3.7 miles (six km), which means that's the distance a person can travel and still find more calories than he or she expends. If an area becomes over foraged, the band quickly senses that and moves the center of its 3.7-mile circle so it reaches into new territory. Such subtle shifts can really build over generations and result in a gradual migration across large landscapes. Many scientists believe this is how humans crossed the North American continent. They did not set out for Kansas. They circled their way there like spinning dancers expanding their range across a floor. A young girl could have lived her entire life within about a fifty-mile radius.

Steve and Rolfe agree with this more conventional theory, but they also think climate changes and extinctions among key fauna, such as mammoths, forced changes in behavior, especially in the Great Plains area, that led to the lengthy migration routes. But even if we stick with the more modest theory of early human migrating patterns, people expended thousands of calories a day on physical activity. In some places, the men hunted for larger game while the women hunted for smaller game and foraged for nuts, roots, and seeds. In other places, women engaged in major hunts or men foraged extensively. For 99 percent of human history people lived as hunter-gatherers. Physical prowess was the gold standard of life. Move, move well, see well, seek well, and your band thrived.

No one wants to do much moving under the midday sun on this particular summer day in Kanorado. When Rolfe tells me that he'd like me to see the other sites—there are three within a half-mile radius—I'm determined to walk this time and ask if we can trek over there. He looks at me politely, points out the prickly bush I'm standing near, and warns me that it can really give a person a razor-sharp cut. I shimmy over a bit, but still insist we should walk.

Too hot, he decides, so I play the polite guest and get back into his truck. We move up a small hill and curve slightly to the right. A second dig comes into view. This time the distinctive dark layer of sediment that Rolfe says marks the period they're investigating stands out markedly in the exposed cliff.

I walk around for a while and look at a few flakes and bones that the diggers have found. I spy a hole and poke my face close to the ground to get a better look.

"Hey, look Rolfe, a burrow."

"Probably a snake," he says, and raises his eyebrows, which feels like a shout coming from someone with his understated personality. "Lots of snakes out here."

I can have all the idealistic ideas I want about moving through the landscape like my hunter-gatherer ancestors, but in reality, I probably couldn't make six kilometers out here on a June day without cutting up my calves on some prickly plant or putting my ignorant face in line with a poisonous snake's front door. I have no idea how to walk this land.

While driving down Route 70, I had noticed some small white seeds floating in the wind. They reminded me of the milkweed I love back East, but since I was moving seventy-five miles per hour in my car, I never did see whether they were the same variety. Precisely because I did not walk here, I did not learn anything about the landscape on my journey. The bands that might have come from Texas, Colorado, and Wyoming would have moved step-by-step and engaged with their local environment in a way that few humans do today. We move our eyes and read screens, newspapers, and books. They moved their bodies and read landscapes. Most of us have become illiterate in that regard.

"It's amazing to think about how durable these people were," Rolfe says. "That to me is one of the most fascinating parts of the story."

It's difficult to think of tribes of people, who lived about forty years less than the average American today, as durable, but they had no vaccines, no antibiotics, no dentists, an inconsistent and limited diet, and lived in an incredibly physically demanding world. They carried big loads, walked huge distances, and often brought down large animals.

As Dr. John Ratey from Harvard Medical School points out in *Spark: The Revolutionary New Science of Exercise and the Brain*, "Our average energy expenditure per unit of body mass is less than 38 percent of that of our Stone Age ancestors. . . . Even if we followed the most demanding governmental recommendations for exercise and logged thirty minutes of physical activity a day, we'd still be at less than half the energy expenditure for which our genes are encoded."

In my eyes, what's equally remarkable is how they used their intimate understanding of their own body mechanics to invent tools that accentuated the power of the arm or channeled the aim of the hand. Probably the supreme example of what I call their "movement intelligence" is the atlatl, a two-part weapon that allows the thrower to heave a lethal dart with accuracy 100 feet or more. For decades, archeologists could not figure out how to re-create a credible reproduction of this device, which humans invented in the Old World about 40,000 years ago and carried with them to the New World around 13,000 to 14,000 years ago.

While Steve and Rolfe have not found any evidence of atlatls at the Kanorado site, scientists know that prehistoric hunters used them to great effect to slay mammoths. A six-foot dart lodges in a two-foot launcher, which they usually made from an antler. For a long time researchers assumed that the dart functioned like a spear, which is rigid. But as former *Outside* magazine columnist Tim Cahill reported in a series of columns, two engineers from Montana State University, Bob Perkins and Paul Leininger, who took an interest in archeology, studied the atlatl puzzle and realized that the dart had to be flexible so it could hold energy and spring free of the launcher.

As Perkins told Cahill, "They didn't have mathematics or a written language, but they understood the concept of physics and wave mechanics and aerodynamics." What they understood was their own bodies and the importance of harnessing and enhancing the power within themselves if they wanted to survive. The engineers figured out the puzzle because they got away from ink and paper and got down-and-dirty in some fields where they tried various designs again and again. They *physically* moved their way to a solution and eventually perfected the Mammoth Hunter Atlatl, which they used to capture the top prize at the 1986 World Atlatl Contest, an event that continues to draw thousands every year.

Clearly I'm not the only one fascinated with the physical activity patterns of our hunter-gatherer ancestors.

The interest isn't that surprising, considering humans spent most of their history in roaming bands; but about 10,000 years ago, groups began settling down, planting seeds, and harvesting a *controlled* food source. For decades scientists assumed that the agrarian lifestyle was a significant step forward on every level for the health and longevity of the average person; but, once again, researchers underestimated the importance of physical movement in the equation.

Farmers did have larger families and more of their children survived to adulthood; but as adults, hunter-gatherers had fewer diseases, stronger bones, a more varied diet, and better teeth. Women in agrarian communities saw the most dramatic reduction in their physical activity levels as they moved indoors for many of their chores, a change that undermined their overall strength. Humans stuck with farm life because domesticated plants and animals meant far more people could live in a much smaller area, a major concern as the human population grew. Neither group had it easy, but the knee-jerk assumption that settling down into a less mobile lifestyle was uniformly good for the human species has proven completely false. We moved in that direction largely because it was the best way to handle a growing mass of people.

Of course the drop off in physical activity for people who shifted from a traditional farming culture to a desk job in a city was even more dramatic and damaging than the shift from wanderer to gardener. Today the farmers near the Kanorado site use chemicals and modern machines to grow their soybeans and other crops. But on those first farms that displaced the nomadic Native American tribes on the Great Plains, the average man put in more than fifty hours of labor a week, and the average woman put in more than forty. During the haying season, the pace became even more intense. They had a vocabulary of action that the average American can no longer understand. Few but the most avid gardeners today know what it means to harrow the fields or to plant 400 celery stalks by hand in one day.

As I think about all the different patterns of human movement on this one square mile of Kansas, the workers from the Kanorado site take a lunch break under the shade of a canopy they've propped up near Rolfe's truck. There are several men and women in their fifties, including Rolfe and Steve, and a handful of graduate students from the University of Kansas where Rolfe teaches and supervises their doctoral studies. I'm much more careful about where I put my feet and where I sit after the snake-hole incident.

The chocolate in my granola has melted. I drink a twelve-ounce bottle of water and still feel thirsty.

Rolfe claims the climate was a bit more temperate when the hunter-gatherers came through here in search of game and water. Today Kanorado gets about ten inches of rain; 10,000 to 13,000 years ago, it was probably as high as thirty.

"There was more game then and things were lusher. There were more trees—cottonwoods, hackberries, willow. There would have been a greater mix of grasses, not just the short grass we see now," he says. "We've even found pelican bones at one of the sites, which suggests there were pools of standing water."

But in the end it wouldn't have looked that much different. The winters wouldn't have been so deep, the summers so hot, but this particular day—in the eighties and clear—could have been a hunter-gatherer kind of day.

Daniel Mandel, Rolfe's twelve-year-old son, bobs and weaves among the workers. He skipped camp so he could come to the dig with his dad. He's already found two important artifacts: a foot bone from a bison and a hand tool. He runs up the hill to try to work the laser station that measures precisely where they uncarth each find. He charges back down. All of the adults sit in the shade and watch him.

"Hey, you know some Pawnee could make sixty miles in a day," Steve says, chatting about the history of ultrarunning among Native American tribes.

"That far?" Rolfe asks.

"Oh, yeah. You should check into that," Steve says, looking at me. "They could just drop and run all day."

"Sounds like my energetic son," Rolfe says. We all laugh. "I guess we sort of untrain them."

2

What Do Our Bodies Want (and Why)?

The History of the Body as Told by the Body

The greatest proof that humans could cover 250 miles (400 km) in a season does not lie in the soil at places like Kanorado. It lies within us. The human physique has changed little in 200,000 years, which means the evolutionary forces that made it possible for prehistoric people to follow migratory mammoth and bison also abide in your feet, ankles, and legs. Modern Americans do not trust or know their bodies the way hunter-gatherers did, but at birth we had as much physical potential to endure long treks as any Kanorado walker, perhaps more. Certainly the average newborn in the U.S. today is taller and heavier than his or her distant forebearers.

For all the complaints about our flawed spine and upright posture, in truth, humans are the ultimate walking machine. To prove the point, just look at the foot. Its long arch distributes weight over the sole and acts as a shock absorber to cushion the body. The Achilles tendon, which gives the leg such a lovely tapered line around the ankle, allows people to raise their full weight off their heel, a motion essential to long-distance running and unique to Homo sapiens. And while apes have opposable big toes, evolution abducted ours, so we lost our ability to grip branches with our feet, but gained better balance for running upright.

For three million years our earliest human ancestors could only walk, not run. But as their bodies evolved to accommodate their upright posture and their need to move more efficiently over long distances, their physiques took on their modern form. If we just continue our tour up the leg, you'll see some of the other marvelous design changes natural selection brought about during that three-million-year tune-up.

Unlike most mammals, humans have separate leg bones below the knee. The fibula moves down into the tibia to stabilize the ankle, which makes it easier to navigate uneven surfaces at high speeds. Of course such scampering requires a finely calibrated sense of balance. Like all mammals, humans have a rectangular-shaped base. In four-legged creatures the four corners are obvious, but in humans the four points rest on the outer margins of the feet to form a much smaller base. This tight center, coupled with the unique angle of our pelvis and femur, means humans expend a lot less energy than our knuckle-walking cousins when they stand, walk, jump, or run.

Above the waist, humans evolved a rib cage that not only supports upright posture but also separates breathing from movement. When reptiles walk they push air from one side of their lungs to the other. They must synchronize their breathing with their gait, which makes long-distance travel impossible. Most mammals also struggle with the separation of the two functions because most four-legged runners, like cats, can take just one breath per stride. The faster they go, the quicker their efficiency drops. The fact they can't pant while they run—a key way to dissipate excess heat—also undermines their endurance.

Ah, but humans, with their specially designed rib cage and diaphragm, can sustain a breathing rate completely independent of their stride. A well-trained athlete can balance his or her oxygen and carbon-dioxide levels for hours.

As the ultimate long-distance travelers, prehistoric people also became adept at carrying things. In relatively recent times, we domesticated animals to carry our burdens, but over very long distances, we could outperform them all; only dogs, hyenas, horses, and some migratory ungulates, like wildebeests, can stick to the hot dusty trail the way we do. Forced to race any of these creatures one-on-one over many days, a supremely fit man would win.

I say "man" deliberately because the two sexes evolved for different types of movement. A woman's hips are on average 7 percent wider than a man's, which makes her better suited for long, slow walks. A man actually requires more power than a woman to move at a moderate pace. If things speed up, as they would in a race or on a hunt, men actually require less energy despite their greater body mass.

For reasons scientists have yet to explain, children under age four really burn up calories when they move, which any parent can tell you makes them pathetic on the hiking trail. Nature offset this problem by making adult humans very efficient carriers. A woman's hip structure makes her especially deft, which explains why females in places like East Africa, where they still transport a lot of water and produce on foot, expend less energy than men when they carry things.

For better or worse, there really is a physical divide between the foragers (women) and hunters (men). The key is to stop valuing one over the other. All the chest-beating hunter-types out there need to know that hunter-gatherer women in many bands foraged for a huge portion of the group's overall calories. Women past childbearing age were especially productive contributors.

Whether they went slow and long or short and fast, our prehistoric ancestors moved. Action generates heat. The better a creature's cooling mechanism, the more energy it can expend. Humans have three million sweat glands. We win. We win by such a large margin that we can track nearly anything into the ground under the noonday heat. The fact we stand upright also means we have less surface area exposed to the sun. Giraffes, antelopes, wildebeests, zebras, gemsboks; all ours if we can just stay at it, often for days, and especially in arid landscapes where most creatures evolved to retain water, which compromises their endurance. Certain prey may pull off greater bursts of speed—humans are actually lousy sprinters—but if they can't cool off as effectively as their pursuer, they will eventually fade. On a continuous run/walk of over sixty miles, a man will lose about twenty pounds of water. Cooling. Replenishing. Outlasting.

Modern people would keel over faster than an antelope in the African sun if they tried to run for days, but that's not because they lack the cooling mechanism of our more robust ancestors; they just haven't developed it. Many existing tribes, including the Khoisan people of South Africa and the Tarahumara Indians of Northern Mexico, who still hunt over long distances on foot, often run down their prey in the hottest part of the day.

Not all animals have a use-it-or-lose-it physique like humans. Bears can hibernate for weeks and still emerge with full strength. A person who laid low for the same amount of time would have problems simply standing up. In the natural world, where movement is a way of life, such immediate adaptability actually proved a strength, because our bodies wouldn't waste energy sustaining muscles we didn't need. It also means we can constantly change what we're good at. Most animals are one-note creatures, but humans can train themselves to excel in a wide range of motions, depending on what circumstances demand.

As a teenager, I used to summer in Cape Cod, Massachusetts, where I'd bike five miles at midday to an outdoor basketball court, play for a few hours, and then bike home. I could never pull off such a feat of endurance today, but at the time I gave it little thought. My body had adapted to a rigorous physical life in the heat.

After back surgery, I had to switch to swimming as my primary exercise. The pool water constantly cools my skin, so no matter how hard I press myself, I never reach the same level of burn. I miss the rivulets of sweat that coursed between my breasts, around my neck, across my brow, and from the back of my knees to my calves. I could feel my body following its own special courses as it relieved me of my heat. I always came home soaked, red-faced, and spent, but after a cool shower, I'd lie down and feel my physical self in a way I never do now in my more tepid middle-aged life.

Sweat is the bowel movement of the skin. Millions of Americans now suffer from a form of constipation because they insist on living the bulk of their lives in climate-controlled environments. Those three million glands not only cool us down, but also purge our body of toxins, like ammonia and uric acid. Humans first evolved in tropical environments where they must have worked up a stinking good sweat every day. I get antsy if my bra gets wet as I walk from the metro to an office downtown. We've compartmentalized perspiration just as we've compartmentalized movement: we give it its allotted hour (and even then only on the days we choose to exercise) and then expect it to disappear.

While Americans recoil at sweat, they've settled down quite comfortably with fat. And why not? Humans have about ten times more fat cells in relation to their body mass than most other animals, which puts us on par with polar bears. For hunter-gatherers who moved around all the time and rarely faced a season of plenty, the human tendency to retain fat was a useful tool, and it remained so even when people settled down on farms about 10,000 years ago because life on those homesteads was also harsh and physically demanding.

As Dr. Henry Lodge, an internist and professor from Columbia University, points out in his book *Younger Next Year,* "In nature, there is no reason to be sedentary except for lack of food." The streambeds dry up. The animals have fled. The plants have shriveled. What do you do? You hole up in the shade and move as little as possible. When we sit in front of a television, we trick our body into thinking it's in precisely that sort of situation: a metabolically passive state because of some outside stress. The biological side of your brain does not understand that you like watching *Seinfeld* reruns. It just knows you're sitting. A lot. Then when you munch on food high in sugar and carbohydrates, your body thinks you've eaten a massive meal—in the wild only something really big and rich could provide that much glucose—so it begins churning out too much insulin, which makes you even hungrier.

Simply snacking while watching a television show for an hour convinces your body that you're both starving and feasting. What a mess. Some forms of sitting are more "active" than others. The TV variety is the worst possible kind because passively watching a screen lowers your metabolic rate to a semi-hibernating state.

To reverse this trend, Americans need to engage in moderate exercise six days a week. Seven would be better, but six will do. The hunter-gatherer daily standard of two to three miles (four to six kilometers) a day has held up for thousands of years and might be a good place to start. The FDA new daily requirements, which suggest sixty to ninety minutes of activity a day, fall right in line with very modest hunter-gatherer patterns, but people and the press have treated them as anything but reasonable. Adults have jobs and families to worry about! Who has ninety-minutes—ninety minutes!—a day to move?

This sense of outrage seems especially egregious if you consider that the ninety minutes can be broken down into many increments over the day and still be effective. In the end, it's less about time than priorities; after all, one of the busiest people on the planet, President Barak Obama, works out regularly and has publicly made the point that physical movement is essential to his mental and emotional health. Before he tackles the financial crisis or latest diplomatic crisis of the day, he gets his blood moving and his mind sharp with physical activity.

If his example is not motivation enough, consider this: some studies have found that an overweight smoker who exercises may have a longer life expectancy than a thin, nonsmoking slacker. People can try the Atkins diet, South Beach Diet, or Weight Watchers, but if they don't move, it won't do them much good. The most powerful determinate of longevity—by far—is exercise. Ever since the 1930s, scientists have known that people who sustain moderate activity levels every day and a low-calorie diet—low enough to make you below weight by American standards but varied and substantial enough for a typical hunter-gatherer—see a 10 to 20 percent increase in life expectancy.

Nature demands movement of all creatures. Clearly we ignore that at our peril. Humans have a tendency to place themselves outside of the wild kingdom, but every physical trait that makes us unique exists in some abbreviated form in another animal: dolphins have remarkable brains; chimpanzees stand upright on occasion; kangaroos use long legs for travel. Of course no other life form combines all of these traits with the same Homo sapiens' flare. Our brain in particular, which burns a monstrous 20 to 25 percent of our total resting metabolism, is so astonishing and has been so deeply impacted by our declining physical life that it warrants its own separate chapter, but right now we must stay with what our bodies can tell us about our capacity to carry out Steve Holen's ambitious vision for us as distance walkers.

So far we have cataloged: springy feet; the heat-saving combination of upright posture, nearly hairless skin, and millions of sweat glands; a huge number of fat cells for when the calories get low; and a diaphragm and lungs that move oxygen and carbon dioxide in and out of our blood stream with crackerjack efficiency. Of course, we mustn't forget our unusual hands, with their power and precision grips that make them ideal for foraging and hunting in a wide variety of habitats.

But this portrait omits one key player that lays the foundation for every move we make and every move any animal makes: the microscopic mitochondria that evolved from a bacterial life form billions of years ago and took up residence in a primitive ancestor about 500 million years ago. Even today your mitochondria are bacterial with their own separate DNA. These mini-engines use oxygen to burn fat or glucose to energize your muscles. They provide the electricity for your house in exchange for a place to live.

Everyone inherits their mitochondria from their mother. Since the mitochondria have their own distinctive DNA, they have become a welcomed marker for scientists to follow as they try to trace the evolution of mankind back in time. Somewhere, some woman had the original mitochondria, which is in all of our bodies today. Of course the canvas has changed over the thousands of years so my mitochondria does not look precisely like yours, but scientists have been able to develop a portrait of the original DNA sequence. They look at slight differences that reflect the passage of time to determine when a given population left Africa, a process called *coalescence.*

Indeed scientists are so good at getting answers about our past from our own bodies that I sense that physical artifacts, like hide scrapers carried from Wyoming, aren't going to matter that much anymore; at least not in terms of providing the key piece of evidence for a hypothesis. Humans now know they evolved in Africa and traveled out of that continent to settle the world. We only had to look within ourselves to discover the news.

How splendid that scientists found the answers to prehistoric peoples' migration patterns in a bacteria that fuels our muscles. When we turn our back on physical activity, we turn away from more than just health. We close our eyes to the story we carry within us.

I confess that while walking the site at Kanorado, I wondered what stories my own fossilized bones would tell archeologists about me if I had lived and died more than 14,000 years ago. Of course they'd be astounded by my size. Amazonian by hunter-gatherer standards. At five feet nine inches and 140 pounds, I would have been as large or larger than the men in my band. I can just picture the notes on the scientist's laptop: *Signs of blunt trauma to the right side of the face, including a cracked eye socket and broken right molar and front incisor; extensive wear and tear on lower vertebrae; improperly healed fracture in left ankle; femur more developed in front than in back—a sign of extensive running over rough terrain; bone density and strength excellent; pelvis markings: one pregnancy.*

Despite the various aches and pains brought about by my athletic injuries, I'm proud to know that if I had died 14,000 years ago, they would have concluded that I'd lived an active life. I had pressed my body long and hard, especially in my youth.

I could have been a Great Plains walker.

3

Physical Grace
The Olympic Center

Of course, today, at age forty-seven, and limited to forty-five minutes of activity a few days a week in a suburban landscape, I probably wouldn't last long in a prehistoric environment, but eager for a modern success story, I knew where to go to find Americans who could: the United States Olympic Center in Colorado Springs, Colorado. I was actually invited to tryout for the Junior Olympic basketball team my junior year in high school, but I failed to break out of the New England regional competition so I never made it to the center. When I finally pull my rental car into the lot, after conquering an airplane seat for four hours, I'm happy I have a far less performance-related agenda. I want to see what can be done with the human body today and what the average person can learn from those gains.

When I meet Bill Sands, a compact, middle-aged man who directs Sports Science at the USOC, he doesn't want to talk about the upper limits of performance, but rather the growing gap between the honed athlete and the American at home.

"The rate of decline in the average person has way outpaced improvements," he says. Back in the early 1900s, when watching sports started to become a major pastime, most Americans worked on farms. The physical differences between the spectator and the athlete were nowhere near as great as they are today.

"When we had a more manual-labor way of making a living, being physical was just part of the day," Sands says, while leaning back in an office chair behind a desk. "[French novelist Emile] Zola, in his book about miners in France [*Germinal*] describes how the men moved so gracefully with no expenditure of extra energy. I mean, look at a cat when it jumps off a table. It looks like water down a hill.

"With the exception of athletes, dancers, and soldiers, everyone else has lost that grace."

Sands himself is a former gymnast and gymnastic coach, who now lifts weights and hikes places like Pikes Peak to stay in shape. While growing up on a farm in Wisconsin, he "pitched a lot of shit" and stayed active from sunrise to sunset. His life changed its trajectory from farming to bioengineering and fitness after he saw some athletes give a demonstration on a trampoline at his high school.

"Wow, I thought, that's incredible. I want to do that."

During our tour of the USOC facility, he showed me a large rectangular-shaped room packed with all sorts of equipment you might see at a military control center: a video that shows 2,000 frames a second; a contraption that measures oxygen consumption. One side of the room focuses on engineering, the other on physiology. Together the technology and the expertly trained advisors, like Sands, provide world-class athletes with minute analyses of what they do right and what they need to do to be better. At one point he showed me a printout of a perfectly performed vault and then the actual movement of a gymnast. Even to my untrained eye, I could see that the athlete was about ten degrees off in his tilt as he cleared the horse.

On one level the facility is incredibly impressive with its ten-lane pool, indoor firing range, extensive weight rooms, and lovely basketball and volleyball courts with a glossy wooden floor. But on another level, it's not that much different than a typical college facility. Financed solely with private funding, the USOC operates on a shoestring. In the end, the 1,000 or so athletes that might be on location at any given time in the year simply have to train their way to excellence. Technology and good equipment can only carry them so far.

When I asked Sands if he thought humans had begun to reach the limits of what they could accomplish on a physical basis in terms of speed and endurance, he said no. "People will continue to break records. I see no end in sight."

From 1924 to 1984, world records improved on average by 30 percent. Progress for male athletes has slowed considerably since then, but among females—well, they continue to improve twice as quickly as men. Of course they had a lot more ground to make up thanks to cultural biases against the sporty girl.

During our interview, Sands received a call from a gymnastic coach asking if he could come to the practice area and provide an audience for the men working on the pommel horse. He figured they'd focus better if people watched. The bare-chested athletes all wore tight-fitting, long Lycra pants that tapered at the ankles. I thought about Sands' comment about physical grace and watched with an admiration that bordered on desire as these young men warmed up on the mats and then tackled the two-handled, four-foot-long apparatus. One of the most difficult rotations in gymnastics, the pommel horse requires great upper body strength, quick hands, and a certain swinging rhythm that can make the best look like a butterfly around a flower and the worst like some klutz trying to clear a fence.

Despite their perfectly muscled upper torsos, the men were clearly still in the earliest stages of their preparation for international competition. Even the former Olympic silver medalist, a tall, slender, dark-haired young man, couldn't pull off a full routine.

"They can only peak for about a week or two," Sands explains, which makes training a very precise science.

I often wonder if our prehistoric ancestors ever thought of their daily movement as "preparation" for something. Did they stretch? Did they "train" for the longer migrations by gradually increasing their mileage day after day? Probably not. For them, movement was not part of some larger goal or competition but an end unto itself. They walked and ran to find food and water and to escape possible predators like the now extinct long-faced bear. They may not have been as finely tuned for one given activity as these world-class gymnasts, but their bodies probably had similar levels of body fat.

A tour group entered the gym and began to applaud after each routine. The collection of twenty plus people were all Caucasian, almost all heavy, except for one middle-aged guy in biker shorts, and awkwardly piled down with cameras, purses, and oversized T-shirts. Their demeanor and noise transformed the setting from an intimate performance into some sort of show. The gymnasts were the zoo animals and the tourists the gawking spectators hoping the lion would roar. They applauded even the most flawed routine, perhaps out of politeness or perhaps because everything the men did was so outside their own realm of physical potential that they just stood in awe.

Here, right before me, stood the divide that Sands had so precisely described. Here, right before me, was grace and the opposite of grace, for which we lack a proper word. How have we allowed ourselves to get to this point and why do we expend so much time and technology on the elite few and yet so little on solving the systemic problems that make it such a struggle for the masses?

The gymnasts fatigued quickly, and the show ended after about thirty minutes. The tour moved on to another part of the USOC facility, and Sands and I returned to his office. I mentioned the tremendous divide between the spectators and the athletes and he nodded his head.

"You know the FDA started out with some Healthy People Goals for 2010, but it became clear that they weren't even going to come close to getting people to change, so they just dumbed the goals down.

"It's an interesting commentary on society and as a species now that we use the brain so much that the body is withering away. Suffering. Dying. This generation is the first time, I understand, that life expectancy will be less than their parents.

"We are in an environment so controlled that it doesn't really challenge us very much. We're not evolving ourselves." [Several recent studies, in particular one funded by the National Institute on Aging in 2005, substantiate Sands' claim that for the first time today's children will have a shorter life expectancy than their parents because of poor lifestyle choices.]

The conversation had become too discouraging so I asked about the growing participation in organized sports, especially among girls. Sands, a former coach and now in charge of sports science at the ultimate sports department, looked disgusted.

"Humans are not built to repeat one task. We're built for variety. And this focus on winning . . ."

He paused and leaned forward.

"I have taken a stopwatch and timed how much *real* activity goes on in organized practices. My daughter plays volleyball, and during a one-hour practice they moved around, well, guess."

"Fifteen minutes," I said.

"Hell, no. Five minutes. It's an astonishing difference. In free play kids move constantly. As a kid on a farm I was out moving all day until dark, but if you watch kids in organized activities the actual time they're moving is not very much. I want to do an official study of that but it's hard because here I deal with the elite."

As adults, only 3 percent of Americans stay in shape by playing team sports, which means our reliance on structured, heavily coached scenarios hardly prepares kids for a future of physical activity that will demand that they be self-motivating and often work out alone.

As I left Sands and his house of superathletes in the late afternoon as a thunderstorm moved into the area, I considered, again, all of the attention lavished on the fringes—the elite performers and the extremely unhealthy—while most of us struggle in the middle with will power, unforgiving work schedules, limited access, money, and more.

Most of us consume too many calories and sit too much. That simple equation pretty much explains why 65 percent of Americans carry around ten or more pounds of excess weight. That number could probably be 75 percent, if I make allowances for the fact that the height and weight charts most doctors use are much too forgiving. If I ever weighed 160 pounds, the upper range of acceptable for my height, I'd be fat.

Terrible things happen to people with such bad habits, including diabetes and heart disease. Obesity has overtaken smoking as the number one cause of death in the United States. There's been so much press about all of this that the only people who don't know about it are either very young or very tuned out. The facts are no longer new, which makes the continual decline seem all that more egregious. We know. As a society we seem paralyzed by indecision about how to fix the problem. Our sedentary culture has the impact of a plague but we treat it like a cold.

Anyone can check on the status of their particular state—the numbers do vary widely—by looking at the State Health Ranking on the American Health

Foundation's website or the National Center for Chronic Disease Prevention and Health Promotion site. Of course it's an imperfect science to measure the general health of a group. Some of the categories include the percentage of uninsured, for example, or measure "leisure" activity, which is such a broad category that it's almost useless, but some hard facts do speak volumes.

In Kansas, for example, home of the hunter-gatherer site, 23 percent of the citizenry are obese compared to 16 percent in Colorado. I could actually see the difference firsthand as I moved through the states, which just underscored for me that a lot more is at work here than simply individual will power. The quest to find out precisely *what* would direct the rest of my research for the next two years.

After the Olympic Center, I stayed at a friend's house in Boulder. I needed a break from all the hours on the road and decided to hike up to the Ouzel Falls in Rocky Mountain National Park. The seven-mile trek at 9,000 feet promised to be a challenge for a flatlander like me, but the falls are clean and trout-filled. While driving out of Boulder along Route 36 towards the trailhead, I passed dozens of cyclists. Some traveled in groups, but many moved alone. The general profile: white, male, age range thirty to fifty. I saw some women, but overall it was a line of Lance Armstrong look-alikes.

All around the Boulder area, home to the University of Colorado, I saw trim, active young people walking, biking, and skateboarding. The overall body language and energy of the town made a marked contrast to the pit stops I pulled into on my way to Kansas, where I often saw entire families of overweight people scarfing down fast food. This place moved.

I opened the windows so the cool, dry morning air circled me. The landscape swept by in soft shades of tan, red, and green. I pulled farther and farther out of town into long stretches where I could use my cruise control, and, still, cyclists showed up alongside the road. As I pulled out of Lyons and into the steep climb toward Estes Park, my car began to struggle. The road curved and cutback, and there were terrible blind spots along the way. I was lucky if I could sustain thirty miles per hour.

I turned off the music so I could concentrate better. The narrow two-lane, two-way road gave cyclists no spare room on the shoulder. They'd suddenly appear around a blind curve, and I'd have a flash of panic as I assessed if I was giving them enough clearance. One guy was pulling a toddler in a carrier on the back of his bike. I started to notice that none of the riders looked playful or joyful, just deeply intent on mastering this enormous 9,000-foot-high mountain pass.

How quickly a Saturday outing of exercise tipped into the extreme. The word "leisure activity" most certainly did not match what these bikers were doing as they moved like members of a cult up a life-threatening road. For them, exercise was not part of the flow of their day, it was a form of self-expression and self-definition that pushed them into deadly places.

Here I was driving in one of the healthiest states in the U.S., and yet I still sensed a terrible imbalance in physical activity patterns. Somehow, even in Colorado, where many people come to be fit, to climb or bike mountains, things are off. Later I learned that Colorado does rank in the top thirteen for states with the highest cycling fatality rates (measured in death rate per million of population).

As Bill Sands reminded me when he mentioned the small amount of time that kids move when they participate in organized sports instead of free play, Americans have started a smoke-and-mirror game. The bikers probably think they're doing something wonderful for their bodies, and on one level they are, but the mental attitude that drives them has little to do with health.

Just as I know firsthand what it feels like to move like water, so, too, do I know the consequences of exercising to the extreme. As a girl, I sustained injuries that I feel every day of my adult life, from my slippery left ankle to the click in my right shoulder, where I ripped some muscles while blocking an inbounds pass. Like the Colorado cyclists, I purged myself with exercise rather than built myself up. In my case, I was a teenager chasing away grief after my father died at age fifty-six. But whatever the reason for the warped attitude, the consequences are the same. It took a life-threatening bike accident to literally and physically realign my own relationship with physical exercise.

By the time I pulled into the parking lot for the Ouzel Falls trail, I felt as though I had survived a harrowing turn around a major highway. I jumped out of my car like a wound spring and began trekking quickly up past the lower falls. The trail is well worn, but I had come early enough to avoid the larger crowds. After just minutes of movement, I felt brisk.

At one point, I passed an overweight boy sprawled on his back in the middle of the path. His father, embarrassed and enraged, was trying to get him moving again. The son even had one foot resting against the knee of the other leg, as though he were reading a novel on a towel at the beach. I swept past and tried to limit the father's shame by not pausing or staring. I heard them arguing behind me as I moved on, the sound of the rushing water on my left, and beads of wildflowers popping up here and there on my right: the iris-like Calypso orchid, harebells, and columbine.

I left behind the bikers, the snake holes, the boy on the trail, and just felt my own legs beneath me, fully strong again after my terrible accident of five years earlier. I increased my pace. I passed the second falls.

This is true grace, I thought, this balance I feel within me, the earth I feel beneath me. Every step I took felt like a celebration, a prayer of gratitude to the forces that shaped me and healed me. I felt like air moving up the mountain. Just air.

4

Flashback

How Did Work Become Sedentary and Physical Activity Become Leisure?

The social history of how Americans slipped into such a sedentary life can begin in many places, but I shall start in my hometown of Hartford, Connecticut. My choice is somewhat personal but hardly arbitrary, since this city on the Connecticut River once lay at the center of cultural life in America. In the nineteenth century such literary lions as Mark Twain and Harriet Beecher Stowe called it home. And some of the largest employers in New England, including the Pope Manufacturing Company, which made bicycles, had their headquarters there. It just so happens that I was raised in a city once full of Beechers and bicycles, two huge players in our nation's journey from a life of physical labor to a life divided between leisure and work.

As a child, I moved through a Hartford famous for its tree-lined avenues and historic homes, many of which still stand. Dutch Elm disease took away the arching branches on many streets, and a struggling local economy, troubled schools, and racial tensions have left many of the splendid neighborhoods in a state of neglect, but evidence of glory remains, like the superb bone structure of an aging beauty's face.

But I did not return to Hartford for the architecture.

I am here because in 1855 Harriet Beecher Stowe's outspoken sister, Catherine (Cate) Beecher, who founded a women's college in Hartford, decided to scold the nation for its declining health in a best-selling book, *Letters to the People on Health and Happiness.* Even though most families still lived on farms prior to the Civil War, an ever-increasing number headed to the cities and to desk jobs that involved no physical labor. This trend led to a whole new pattern of health problems, including unusually high rates of depression, anxiety, nervous disorders, back problems, and stomach ailments.

"Many men avoid healthful pursuits as less honorable," Beecher wrote. "Instead they prefer to remain shut up in study, office, or store, which overworks the brain and leaves the muscular system run down for want of vigorous exercise and fresh air."

As for women, well the majority of them "are systematically educating the rising generation to be feeble, deformed, homely, sickly and miserable," she declared with typical Beecher authority.

To understand the weight of the Beecher name in mid-nineteen-century America, think Martha Stewart, Bill Moyers, or even Kennedy. Cate's father, Lyman Beecher, was one of the most dramatic preachers in New England. Her brother, Henry Ward Beecher, followed in his father's footsteps and made a mark as a minister on a national scale. And, of course, Harriet Beecher Stowe's book *Uncle Tom's Cabin* was one of the most influential American novels of the nineteenth century.

As for Cate herself, the eldest of the eleven remarkable Beecher children, by the time she published *Letters to the People* she had already founded the women's college I alluded to earlier, the Hartford Female Seminary, as well as the Western Female Institute in Cincinnati, Ohio. She had also published another big-selling book, *Domestic Economy*, which urged women to take their household duties as seriously as men take their careers.

When a Beecher spoke, Americans listened.

Cate had a particular passion for her subject in *Letters to the People* because, like myself, she was driven to write her book after battling back problems, which left her so disabled that she had trouble walking. She tried several doctors over many years. They prescribed various drugs and lots of rest, but nothing worked. She began to look back at her healthy childhood in Litchfield, Connecticut, and tried to piece together what made it such a vigorous time in her life. She decided it came down to two things: fresh air and exercise.

"The purity and strength of the whole body is dependent on the *proper exercise of the muscles*," she concluded.

Cate left Hartford in 1832 to found a college in Cincinnati devoted to training new teachers for Western schools. She didn't last long in St. Louis—her New England candor did not go over well with the locals—so she returned East in 1838. As an unmarried woman with no children, she had few resources and even with the income from her writing, she had limited means, so she began staying with various relatives, "like a trunk without a label," as her witty sister Harriet claimed in a letter to a sibling.

But her travels also gave her the opportunity to research the health of American women across the country from Wisconsin to Vermont. She began to circulate formal questionnaires among the ladies in various towns and to tally the results, which she published in *Letters to the People*.

"In the first place, the *standard of health* among American women is so low that few have a correct idea of *what a healthy woman is*." Cate lamented the poorly ventilated houses, the sharp decline in physically engaging domestic chores, and the restrictive clothing women felt obliged to wear. Then she listed her disturbing results:

"*Milwaukee, Wis.* Mrs. A. frequent sick headaches. Mrs. L. poor health constantly.

Essex, VT, Mrs. S. very feeble, Mrs. G. quite feeble.

New Bedford, Mass., Mrs. B. pelvic disorders, and every way out of order. Mrs. J. W. pelvic disorders.

Hartford, Conn. I can think of only one [healthy woman] . . ."

And so she continued for pages.

Of course many of these women's problems stemmed from delivering babies in unsanitary conditions. And the prejudices that kept women out of classrooms and careers and undervalued the work they did perform on the home front certainly contributed to the high rate of depression. But, as Cate Beecher knew, these factors had always been there, and yet the collective physical decline continued at an alarming rate. It had to be the shift toward a sedentary life, she concluded, and the tendency to close houses so tightly no one could take a clear breath.

She called for every American to "take a great deal of exercise; breathe only pure air, both by day and night; bathe often; never exercise the brain more than five or six hours a day." This was radical stuff in 1855, in part, because the concept of leisure as we know it was still in its infancy.

In the eighteenth century, Americans lived such labor-intensive lives that they had little spare time and much of that was filled with communal obligations, like church, or, perhaps, a harvest festival. By the early 1800s, some sports, in particular boxing, fox hunting, horse racing, and gymnastics, began to take hold, but these were hardly things the average person pursued.

The rise of the desk worker and the number of labor-saving devices for women at home created a space in the day that hadn't existed for most people before. Cate herself had the peculiar idea of building Temples of Health in each community to help fill that time. She envisioned a team of doctors always on hand in the center of town at a place where people could come to listen to music, get a physical evaluation, and then engage in exercises prescribed by the medical staff. She had to stretch for answers because games like basketball hadn't been invented yet and the idea of going for a recreational run was just not part of the collective public consciousness.

I thought about all of this as I walked across Asylum Avenue in Hartford to reach the Connecticut Historical Society, which has lots of material on the Beechers. The rain smacked the pavement so hard the rebounding drops wet my leg mid-calf. Police had closed off the street for the Hartford Marathon so everything was oddly quiet. A handful of volunteers, umbrellas in hand, suddenly stopped talking as a tall African man came over the rise running at an incredible clip. After looking at a map in *The Hartford Courant* the day after the race, I learned that the Kenyan was near the finish of the marathon, but in the gray of that moment, he looked incredibly fresh and ran from one end of the block to the other faster than I could if that's all I had to run. A motorcycle with a cameraman rode less than two feet from him. It was clear he was a professional runner and so far ahead that no one else came into view between when I saw him and the time I entered the historical society.

Ninety minutes later I emerged to find the street awash with people in colorful sneakers and shorts. Some headed away from the city, others headed toward it, depending on which part of the loop they were on. All looked exhausted. One person had taken his shoes off and walked the last few miles barefoot. A few overweight people struggled past. I heard a volunteer or two shout some encouragement, but overall it was a grim, determined bunch at the twenty-plus mile mark of a long race.

Perhaps Cate's Temple of Health wasn't so weird after all. At least she included music and thought of exercise as something you did to relieve stress and to build strength, not as some proving ground. The idea of making a living as a professional long-distance runner would have been as alien to nineteenth-century Americans as, well, their farm life feels to us.

But even as I concede this, I know in the back of my mind, before my back injury, I had often thought of training for a marathon. I liked the challenge and camaraderie, and longed for the indescribable sensation of being in superb shape. I realize as a former college athlete and extreme competitor, who aspires to find a more balanced relationship with physical activity, I contain within me the whole continuum of the American relationship with movement, part leisure, part challenge, part chore, part celebration. Physical activity has become infinitely more complex than something we just do for survival.

Before stumbling upon the Hartford Marathon, I had taken a tour of Harriet Beecher Stowe's house on Farmington Avenue, where she lived from 1873 until her death in 1896. I wanted to walk where Cate Beecher had walked, on the steep, narrow steps of her famous sister's house. I thought about Cate's bad leg as I made my way down the backstairs to the kitchen. It's a tight Victorian home stuffed with period furniture and many of Harriet's remarkable paintings of local wildflowers. Visitors can see Mark Twain's house, with its striking brickwork, out the back window. The great American humorist and Harriet were neighbors for decades.

I knew about Twain, but not about many of the other illustrious people who shared this 140-acre area known as Nook Farm. As I read the biographies of Harriet's various neighbors, I came across a photograph of Joseph Roswell Hawley, former U.S. senator and Connecticut governor, who had a house just down the hill by the railroad tracks.

I scanned his biography and saw that Hawley had helped organize the U.S. Centennial Exhibition in Philadelphia in 1876, a World's Fair-type of extravaganza. What an incredible piece of serendipity. Here was a person who linked the two primary characters in my Hartford story: a Beecher, who was one of the first to warn Americans about the health consequences of a sedentary lifestyle, and the bicycle, the first real answer to the need for general recreation.

The Centennial Exhibition Hawley helped organize had a display of British-made bicycles, which Albert Pope, son of an eighth-generation lumbering family in New England, saw at the fair. On the spot, Pope put in an order for thirty of the contraptions and made up his mind he would get into the business of building them himself.

And so began the saga behind an object that transformed leisure unlike anything Americans had ever seen.

The bicycle that enthralled Pope looked little like the ones we ride today. Built in England and called a velocipede, the front wheel was enormous, the back tire tiny, the wheels hard as stone, and the ride extremely bumpy. But Pope ordered them anyway. When he went looking for floor space for his new factory, he came across the Weed Sewing Machine Company in Hartford, which had seen a dramatic drop-off in business after the Civil War and had some empty warehouses and plenty of machinists looking for work.

When the wind came off the Connecticut River, Harriet Beecher Stowe could hear the machines at the Pope Manufacturing Company. Cate Beecher herself would have heard the background clamor when she came for one of her lengthy visits. There's no record of what Cate thought of this new-fangled invention, but I have to think she must have approved of anything that encouraged the masses, including women, to get outside for exercise and fresh air.

Initially, Pope's seventy-pound bicycles appealed only to the well-to-do adventurous man who could join a club that had a riding track, membership fees, and even a uniform. As the Connecticut Bicycle Club—probably the first wheeling club in the U.S.—stated in its 1879 handbook, "The uniform shall be a sack coat, knee breeches, stockings and polo cap with visor, all of the dark green color and a white helmet hat." Members had to pay a $15 annual fee.

But then in the late 1880s, an Irish veterinarian looking to make a softer ride for his ailing son invented the pneumatic tire, which is filled with air. This invention coupled with better gears, tires of equal size, and foot brakes transformed the bicycle into something that nearly anyone could ride. Advances in making nickel into steel alloy also meant lighter frames. By the 1890s, hundreds of thousands of Americans were riding the Pope Manufacturing

Company's twenty-two-pound Columbia bicycle. In just two decades, Albert Pope's hunch had helped make him the biggest employer in New England.

While at the Connecticut Historical Society, I flipped through advertisements for the Columbia bicycle, which featured women in flowing skirts riding leisurely through the countryside. By the turn-of-the-century, women accounted for at least a third of all bicycle sales, a statistic that would have made Cate Beecher blush with excitement.

So the humble bicycles shoved in our garages and garden sheds set in motion a revolution in recreation in the United States. Items like women's bike bloomers, a loose-fitting pair of pants, opened the door for more sensible clothing. For the first time large numbers of middle-class men participated in organized races; the best often trained so seriously that pundits in the press worried if sport was creating monster humans. And the fiercest competitors, like the great African American wheeler Marshall Major Taylor, became national celebrities. Millions of Americans of all ages and both sexes sat on the seats of their new machines and rode right into a whole new physical life centered on a sharp divide between work and leisure and which glorified superior performers.

The bicycle had become so common that Harriet's neighbor Mark Twain could write an essay in 1888 about his own attempts to conquer the beast and know that most readers would be in on the joke.

"I thought the matter over, and concluded I could do it," he began in "Taming the Bicycle." He gets a package deal at the Pope factory that includes a bicycle and individual lessons on how to ride. A Laurel & Hardy routine ensues as he runs down his instructor several times.

"The bicycle had what is called the 'wabbles,' and had them very badly," Twain concluded. "Try as you may, you don't get down as you would from a horse, you get down as you would from a house afire. You make a spectacle of yourself every time."

Despite his many travails, Twain did notice the superior muscles of his instructor, so he pressed on. In the end, he crashes into a cabbage wagon, blaming his own poor steering and the state of the bumpy road.

"I had been familiar with that street for years, and had always supposed it was dead level; but it was not, as the bicycle now informed me."

Twain hit on a touchy subject for bicycle riders and for the Pope Manufacturing Company itself: the nation needed better roads for bicycling to succeed across the country. As part of the Good Roads Movement in the 1890s, Pope himself paid to have some sample pavement laid down in Hartford so riders could experience what it felt like to ride on a smooth surface. Millions of bicycle owners proved a formidable force for change, and in 1893, before the first car ever got off an assembly line, Congress decided the federal government had to get into the road-building business.

Despite the huge rise in bicycle sales and the dramatic increase in organized sports teams in colleges, many other strong voices joined Cate Beecher in sounding the alarm about the nation's collective physical decline. If I move beyond Hartford to Boston, I bump into an indignant Ralph Waldo Emerson, a hard-walking Henry David Thoreau, and an appalled Oliver Wendell Holmes, who claimed that "such a set of black-coated, paste-complexioned youth as we can boast in our Atlantic cities never before sprang from the loins of Anglo-Saxon lineage."

"Physical depletion among middle class males reached epidemic proportions in 1900," says author Carolyn Thomas de la Pena in *The Body Electric: How Strange Machines Built the Modern American.*

"The state of pervasive weakness created more than a physical change in American culture; it also created a cultural change, as white middle class men attempted to build muscle in emulation of new vigorous heroes like Harry Houdini . . . and Teddy Roosevelt, fellow white collar men who embodied the self made confidence and physical strength they lacked."

The collective decline in health, especially among men, led to a lot of hand wringing about the superiority or inferiority of civilized societies. Newspapers ran tales of Native Americans who could pull back bowstrings that white American males could barely budge, and day laborers who could lift huge amounts of weight while the softened office worker could just stare. Some argued that in the new industrial world physical fitness counted for nothing, and a muscled man was the mark of a savage, but others—the majority—feared for the safety of the nation.

How could a country effectively defend itself if its young men couldn't even haul hay?

Through most of the nineteenth century, the term "physical education" referred to hygiene, but as the average citizen became more and more concerned about the country's fitness, educators began to put the physical into P.E. Men like Dr. Dudley Allen Sargent, director of the gym program at Harvard University in the 1870s and founder of the Sargent School of Physical Training in Cambridge, Massachusetts, in the 1880s, insisted that what machines had taken away they could now give back in spades. At Harvard he installed fifty-two contraptions, some the precursors to contemporary fitness equipment like the StairMaster, and had each entering freshman go through his paces. Dr. Sargent or one of his assistants would identify the physical weaknesses of each student and then map out a fitness program that he had to stick to throughout his years at Harvard. This sort of regimented, measured approach to exercise marked a whole new way of seeing the human body. This was beyond simple manual labor, beyond leisure, and into fitness as a science.

The Sargent School became Sargent College (now part of Boston University), which my mother attended after World War II. She majored in physical therapy and physical education, a program of study that Sargent himself had put into place. Since a woman in the 1940s had few career choices, the fact my mother could aspire to be a physical-education teacher shows how far American thinking had come with regard to encouraging activity among girls and fitness in schools. Of course sexism was rampant, and boys were far more apt to play organized sports, like baseball and basketball, but things had still improved dramatically from Cate Beecher's time.

My mother eventually taught physical education, among other subjects, in Hartford's public schools. So my circles continue to twirl around my hometown.

By the time I entered high school in the 1970s in the Hartford area, enough had changed for girls that I was able to push my physical limits in just about any sport I chose to pursue. The line of spectators at our events was pretty thin, but if I wanted to compete, if I wanted to explore the science of my own body, the possibilities were endless right up to the Olympic level.

During the same visit I landed in the middle of the Hartford Marathon, I drove around to some of my favorite outdoor parks, where I used to play basketball for hours. The courts used to be packed, and since only winners got the next game, only the best stayed on for long. There weren't many young, white girls playing the game back then, but the courts were always moving. Today most of these public spaces are empty either because kids spend all their time in organized sports or because the parks simply aren't that safe anymore.

As a girl, I knew enough never to play in Pope Park, founded by bicycle kingpin Albert Pope. The African American kids from the rough North End used to play there (and produced some world-class players, I must add), but a blonde would never have been welcomed. Today, Hispanic families have moved into the neighborhood, and the North End crowd often battles with the newcomers. Few go into that space at night.

Pope created the park so the workers at his factory could have a nice open space during their off hours. He wanted them to walk, listen to music, and, of course, to bicycle. But like so many public spaces in America, Pope Park has become a place where unstructured play and casual outings are no longer possible. One of the great under-told stories in the physical-fitness saga is the role of the declining use of public parks for casual play. Near my home most of the fields require a permit before a group can use the field. If my young daughter brought some friends to a local field for a pick-up game of kickball, city officials would chase them away. A kid is either on a team and training or sitting on the sidelines, or worse, in front of a screen at home.

Besides my parents, few things shaped my character as profoundly as my experiences as a white girl playing pickup basketball games with black males in the Hartford area. They patronized me and called me honey and didn't include me in the flow when I was in a game, or they shunned me altogether and refused to acknowledge that I was in line to play "next." I kept coming back, because I knew they—not the backboard in my suburban driveway—held the key to really learning the game. I don't know why I was so obsessed with moving with a ball at such an early age or why I risked so much to belong where I would never belong, but I could shoot and I was fast and played real defense—a rarity in street hoops. I never shined against the backdrop of their superior strength and agility, but I had "game" and they came to respect that.

The only holdouts were the physically insecure white men who came to play. Well-acquainted with prejudice, the black players began to take me under their wing, and the strongest units would purposely include me, challenge the team with the white players, and then set me up for wide-open shots again and again.

"Ohhhh, how 'bout that," they'd taunt and laugh in the white guys' faces.

Today I work for myself, in part, because of what I learned on those city courts. Mastering the nuances of the social interplay, mastering the way the ball is supposed to roll around in your hand when you dribble, took discipline, focus, and a clear sense of myself. I knew where I wanted to bring my body and I took myself there. I know where I want to be as a writer and I'm taking myself there with this very line.

Public spaces and free play gave me these things, something my daughter will probably never know.

But my Hartford story doesn't end here, because Pope's story is not finished. For a man who had such an enormous impact on the city in the nineteenth century, there's little left to mark his passing. No tourist center, like the one on Nook Farm for Twain and Stowe, to celebrate the central role he once played in Connecticut's capital.

The Pope Manufacturing Company used dozens of people to craft one Columbia bike, an inefficient production process that their competitors used to price them out of the market in the early twentieth century. Pope had already shifted his attention elsewhere anyway, toward the next machine that would transform not only American leisure but also every aspect of American life: the automobile.

The young mechanical wizard Hiram Percy Maxim teamed up with Pope and used the bicycle mechanics and factory space to produce one of the first commercial cars in the U.S., the 1897 Mark III Stanhope. Powered by batteries that made up nearly half of its 18,000-pound weight, the Mark III could reach speeds of thirty miles per hour. It rolled out with great fanfare on the streets of Hartford, inspiring a visiting British reporter to write that Connecticut was the "greatest center of activity in the automobile industry today."

But Pope's cars didn't take off the way he expected them to because— to his surprise—smelly, gasoline-driven automobiles proved more popular, practical, and cheaper to produce. The Pope mobiles, which came in an array of models, catered to the elite buyer. The industrialist Henry Ford figured out if he produced one basic model and built his factory close to the steel manufacturers in the Midwest, his company could churn out cars much faster and more cheaply than anything Pope had coming out of his factory.

By the time the Model T rolled off the assembly line in 1908, Pope was out of business.

One of the books I found at the Connecticut Historical Society had a photograph of President Teddy Roosevelt riding with Alfred Pope in a Pope-manufactured car down the streets of Hartford. The year: 1902.

How many things come together in that one shot: The paved roads; the car instead of the carriage (or bicycle!); the president who established the National Park system riding in the very invention that would make access to those parks possible, but also undermine many an American's desire to engage with those remarkable landscapes from anywhere but the safety of their automobiles. The car would simultaneously open up the entire continent, but close us off from our physical selves. We would never engage with our bodies or our public spaces in the same way again.

5

Moving on the Job Today
Assembly Lines in Pennsylvania

After reading about assembly lines, I decided to drive out Route 30 in Pennsylvania, past the few remaining farms and endless miles of nondescript development, to get to a long, low building—the Utz Potato Chip factory in Hanover—so I can see firsthand what it means to move the human body not to survive, not for leisure, but purely as a means of production; profit and efficiency, not fitness and pleasure, rule here. In the factory lobby, a young, narrow-faced woman with brightly colored orange curls that fall past her shoulders introduces herself as Kris Shakely, my guide for the morning and Utz's occupational nurse.

At our first stop overlooking the machines, women in blue aprons pick burnt potato chips off a conveyor belt. More than three thousand pounds of chips rumble by every hour. In my perch behind a glass panel about six feet above their heads, I can feel an intense vibration rising through my feet as though the building has a cold and is shivering.

"We move the chips with vibrations so they won't break," Kris says.

I say nothing for almost a minute and just let the movement of the machines fill me. There's so much controlled energy in this place from the potato-chip slicer to the conveyor belt rolling bags at a methodical but relentless clip.

"I've done all of the jobs here," Kris says. "I picked for two hours and I tell you I've never been so grateful in my life that I went to college. I get motion sick watching those chips go by. They said you get used to it."

When most Americans think about the history of the assembly line they think of Henry Ford, who, of course, used it to keep costs down and his Model T affordable for the masses. Ford actually borrowed the idea of assigning workers specific, repetitive tasks along a carefully laid-out line from the meat-packing industry, so his approach was hardly new. The real genius of the Ford Motor Company lay in the fact that its founder thought he could produce something as big as a car for a lot of people for very cheap. When he opened his business in 1903, the factory produced a few thousand cars, but by 1914 the line made a record 230,000 Model Ts, each cheaper than the last. The original models went for about $700, but Americans could get the 1914 edition for as little as $400.

There are darker numbers behind this success story, including a 900 percent turnover rate among Ford employees in 1913. Just watching the Utz potato-chip pickers for fifteen minutes gave me a very clear understanding why no one wanted to work nine-hour days on a Ford assembly line performing the same, narrowly defined task. A potato chip may weigh less than an ounce, but try scanning, leaning, and snatching for even thirty minutes and suddenly weight is no longer the problem. Even minute movements become unbearable if you have to repeat them enough.

Ford got around the huge attrition rate by doubling wages. Utz tries to get around the repetitive motion injuries by shifting the blue-apron women to a new station every thirty minutes. They can start the day as pickers then move to boxing, where they must swoop three large bags of chips off the belt and into a box.

"There's no way to slow the machines," says Kris, "and the bags have to go into the box a certain way." A woman at one of the bagging stations turns and waves to Kris and startles me with her smile. Kris, who seems so out-of-place here, gestures back.

"Do you know her?"

"Oh, yes. I know them all."

I ponder the fact that the occupational nurse "knows them all" as I watch the baggers. I notice that some pinch the three bags together between their right and left hands and drop the chips into the box, while others use their right arms to swing the bags toward their bodies—the "right" way to do the task.

"We try to teach them proper technique but it's hard to redo form."

I think I'd be a pincher myself. The bags look so airy and easy to swing around, but clearly the repetition is taxing. Kris says the women pair up with a trusted co-worker at the bagging station and stick with that person for years. I notice some people wearing only white—temps; none of them have blue-aproned partners.

After my tour past the pickers, baggers, blade changers, spicers, and salters, I meet Kris's colleague, Jeff Weinman, a hefty middle-aged white man and an occupational therapist from the local hospital, who often works with Utz employees. He's drawn up a precise outline of the physical requirements for each job on the floor. He puts new employees through a series of tests to see which jobs they can handle. Can they stand for eight or nine hours a day? Can they move skids loaded with boxes or shift eighty-pound bags of salt?

"We don't just randomly stick someone in a new position," Jeff says.

I mention Frederick Winslow Taylor to them, a name that flies over Kris's head and brings just a faint sign of recognition from Jeff, which is no surprise. I had never heard of Taylor either until I began studying movement in detail, but Americans can credit this early twentieth-century time-management expert with the way they get their McDonald's hamburgers, the way their BlackBerries help them organize their days, and the way Jeff diagrams the physical requirements for a given factory job right down to the height of a skid or the pace of the conveyor belt.

As Robert Kanigel, director of writing at the Massachusetts Institute of Technology (MIT), says in his book *The One Best Way: Frederick Winslow Taylor and the Enigma of Efficiency*, Taylor "bequeathed a clockwork world of tasks timed to the hundredth of a minute, of standardized factories, machines, women, and men. He helped instill in us the fierce, unholy obsession with time, order, productivity, and efficiency that marks our age."

Raised in Philadelphia, Taylor left his middle-class life as a young man to work as a laborer in the steel industry in the late 1800s. He eventually worked his way into management because of his remarkable ability to break a task down, identify the "one best way" to perform it, then show all of the other laborers the technique.

He looked at things like how large a shovelhead should be for a man to move coal most efficiently. Does the answer change if he's moving gravel or sand instead? Taylor took out his measuring tape and his stopwatch and arrived at specific, repeatable numbers. For example, he concluded that a worker using a shovelhead that held 21.5 pounds of coal would have the largest pile at the end of the day.

With speed and productivity his primary objectives, Taylor—or one of his disciples—began applying his scientific time-management formulas to manufacturing plants throughout the United States. In 1913, the year before Ford sold a record 230,000 cars, Taylor went into a competing Packard plant and reduced the number of workers on the production line by half, transforming that company into a legitimate threat to Henry's Model Ts.

Of course such steely-eyed draconian strokes hardly enamored him to the average laborer. While testifying about his time-management work before a Congressional panel in 1912, he went into detail about shovels and piles.

"You have told us the effect on the pile," observed Congressman John Q. Tilson, "but what about the effect on the man?"

I think of that quotation as I listen to Kris Shakely talk about the Utz truckers and route salesmen. They must hop in and out of their vehicles all day long, bouncing on knees, straining backs, hauling boxes.

"We get the largest turnover in these jobs," Kris says, which surprises me, because at least they're outside and have some control over their own time. But they are also alone most of the day. There's no blue-aproned teammates out there.

I lean over the edge of a conveyor belt loaded with three-foot-high boxes packed with bagged chips. The rollers go on and on for at least a half mile. Other than Kris and me, there are no other people in sight, just the sound of productivity, the sound of efficiency.

By the early 1900s, with Taylorism in full swing, engineering had become the largest profession in the United States after teaching. The end result: all the things that bring an Utz potato-chip bag to your local 7-Eleven.

But to really complete the picture of Americans' changing relationship between their bodies and their jobs, I need to reach back even further than Taylor, to the first serious scientist of human movement, the Frenchman Etienne-Jules Marey.

Jeff Weinman at Utz had some knowledge of Taylor, but almost no one knows of this small, bearded European who made major contributions to photography then used his newfound technical equipment to study the laws of movement in animals, humans, water, air, indeed just about anything that shimmied and shaked.

"From the invisible atom to the celestial body lost in space, everything is subject to motion," Marey wrote. "It is the most important characteristic of life."

The son of a wine steward and schoolteacher's daughter, Marey actually wanted to be an engineer, but his parents pushed him into medicine. He fused the two professions by building machines to help him answer his medical questions about movement. He wanted to "express the most fleeting, most delicate, and most complex movements which no language could ever express," he wrote.

First he looked inward at circulation, respiration, and the human heart. Inspired by the melograph, a machine that moved spokes over specially marked paper to play music, he created the first polygraph, which had a long, thin arm with a needle on the end that responded to a patient's pulse and left a neatly drawn line on a piece of moving carbon paper. For the first time, someone had a visual graph of a "normal" heart pattern. For a hundred years, doctors throughout the world used the polygraph and many of Marey's other inventions for measuring internal functions.

Next he went to work measuring external human movements. By the 1870s, photography had advanced enough that many people had taken pictures of humans walking up stairs, of horses at full gallop, or a woman pouring water into a sink, but no one could show an uninterrupted sequence of images. Marey tried pasting stamp-sized shots onto a wheel known as a zoetrope, which when spun gave the viewer the impression that the image was moving. The zoetrope images were not only primitive but also very labor-intensive to produce. Marey had to take dozens of photographs of something in motion then develop the individual shots, organize them in a credible sequence, and then paste them one-by-one onto the hand-held contraption.

At the same time that Marey wanted a more detailed way to chronicle human movement, a French astrophysicist, Jules Janssen, wanted a way to track stars. He crafted a photogun, which used the new soft Kodak roll film invented in America (instead of wet plates). He took much faster and more precise photographs than anyone had ever taken. Marey took Janseen's gun and made it even speedier and more accurate. Armed with his new machine, a staff, and financial backing from a French government in a panic over the health of a nation of men that had just lost the Franco-Prussian War, Marey went to work.

He painted the background of the photography studio black. He even dressed his primary subject, the assistant Georges Demeny, in black then put strips of white tape on his knee and other key joints. When Marey took a picture of Demeny walking, only the movement of the tape showed up, which allowed Marey to pare it all down to just the mechanics of the leg, the angle of the torso, the swing of the arm.

In other pictures he allowed Demeny to move naturally in regular sports clothes and then ran the sequence of photographs all together so that there might be eight or nine images of Demeny in various stages of motion overlapping each other on one page. This was photography just before cinema; the closest anyone had come to actually filming a person in action.

Much of Marey's work had been lost and forgotten until a Canadian scholar, Marta Braun, uncovered boxes of his negatives in the 1990s. Even to my media-savvy eyes, I feel Marey's photographs capture the energy inherent in the human body in a way that even the most advanced cinema today fails to do.

I especially like the sequence of images of Demeny walking in his white gymnastic pants and shirt and small French cap. The jumble of leg images underscores how complicated something as simple as a forward step can be and how much snap there is in the knee, how much spring in the foot. His head is very erect and his trim torso barely alters its angle with each step, like a soldier marching. The right arm swings and swings with each sequence and forms an "L" on his side. I sense the upright nature of our bodies and the elegant lines of a physically fit person. Marey captured the fundamental grace of the average man.

He also made the French government very happy by coming up with all sorts of very specific insights about the ideal weight for a soldier's backpack, the quickest walking pace a man can sustain before breaking into a run (seventy paces a minute), and the best way to lift heavy objects (bend at the knees).

When the Americans trounced the French in track and field at the 1900 Olympics, Marey's government turned to him for answers, and he used his photography studies to show that the Frenchmen were in better shape but had lousy technique. The Americans knew how to lean into a hurdle at the proper time or how to use their second leg to give them momentum as they swung over the high jump. While Marey remained completely immersed in the study of movement, other scientists and physical-education professionals began applying his findings to sport and industry. Demeny went on to found France's first comprehensive physical-education programs, and men like Frederick Winslow Taylor looked to Marey's results to show that every aspect of every job could be measured and assessed for the proper way of doing things.

It's hard for us to understand to what extent Marey's work opened up a whole new way of seeing and measuring the human body. Scientists began to identify norms for all sorts of internal and external movements. Athletes began to look at their own bodies as machines that could be trained in precise, performance-enhancing ways. Even artists, enthralled by the new sense of time and movement expressed in Marey's photographs, which showed any given "moment" as actually a series of smaller events, began playing with human movement in their paintings. Marcel Duchamp's "Nude Descending a Staircase," is the most famous example of the Cubism that Marey's work inspired.

While looking for a way to put a more human face on this pioneer in the study of human movement, I came across a firsthand account of a person who had heard Marey give a lecture at a theater in Sorbonne.

"People came to listen to Marey explain the true artistry of the mechanisms of life, the laws of ancient and modern dance, the movements of animals; the progression of fish, gaits of horses, and flights of birds and insects. He was a charming lecturer, one who spoke spiritedly of gymnastics and aviation and who celebrated with emotion the wings of pigeons and dragonflies."

When Kris Shakely tells me at the Utz manufacturing plant that all of the trucks come in at noon to load up and "it's like a ballet," I think of Marey's vision of animal movement as "true artistry." But when truck drivers sit for hours every day and perform repetitive lifting that hurts their knees and backs, it's not a proper dance. The whole factory makes me feel how much we've violated the contract we have with our bodies in most workplaces and I just want to leave.

On my way out, Kris tells me she thinks the blue-aproned workers complain too much about small aches and pains and that the prison workers she interacted with at her last job at a concrete company never whined.

"Those men were so grateful to have a job that they'd work through anything."

I want to remind her that she herself was exhausted after just two hours of picking chips, but I don't. Humans have a remarkable knack for adapting to whatever a situation demands of them. Americans have come to accept work conditions in offices and in factories that require them to repeat the same motion day after day. It might be typing or salting potato slices, but it's definitely not good for their bodies. At least at Utz the workers shift stations every thirty minutes, a concession that men like Henry Ford rarely made.

I sit in my car for at least fifteen minutes after leaving the factory. I watch some yellow linden leaves spin circles around the field in front of me. Kris kindly gave me a huge box stuffed with various Utz chips and pretzels for my teenage daughter Julia, who was incredibly excited that I was visiting such a "fun" assembly line. Of course, after watching the blue-aproned workers, I know there's no such thing as a "fun" assembly line, something I understood but never felt before I came. I mean, really, how could I stomach buying anything, from chips to cars, if I thought too hard about how it's made and who must abuse their bodies to make it for me?

I try to shake that feeling as I drive away, but it's very, very hard.

I have one more stop on my road trip: the Harley-Davidson motorcycle plant about thirty minutes away in York, Pennsylvania. All of my research into bicycles, the paving of America, the impact of the automobile (and other gas-powered transportation) on people's physical habits and the shift away from brawn to brains and machines in the workplace make the Harley-Davidson factory too compelling to miss.

It's a huge, dark, noisy, oily smelling place. For the first half of our tour, I don't see a single person doing a job—just blue lasers cutting parts and heavy machines moving objects along a conveyor belt. Our guide, Jeff, a white-haired, middle-aged intelligent man, speaks to us through special headphones because the background din is too great to hear anyone more than a few feet away.

The air begins to make me asthmatic, and I feel jittery because of the huge number of moving objects all around me. The athlete in me wants to respond like a defender in a basketball game. There are weird little booths here and there framed by strips of orange plastic. I can see the faint silhouette of men working at computer stations at several of these islands.

Just when I'm about to call it quits because of the stressful environment, the people-driven assembly line comes into view. Like a primary artery, a set of twenty-four stations with two people at each station (one on either side of the motorcycle) runs down the center of the factory floor. Most of the workers are white men with big paunches and strong forearms, but there are also a few women, all dressed in T-shirts, jeans, and functional sneakers. They pull long tubes with some sort of instrument on the end and bolt some part into place as the bike goes by.

The factory produces 850 motorcycles a day. The line moves six feet per minute. Like the potato chip factory, there's no sense that anything is moving rapidly here, just relentlessly.

The final station Jeff shows us has two tall white guys wearing jeans, T-shirts, and bandanas on their heads, test-riding sample motorcycles coming off of the line.

"They have the complete authority to accept or reject a bike," Jeff says, then explains they base their judgments on sound, vibrations, and a general intuition that comes from years of experience.

"This is not an entry-level job," he says, with a slight laugh and a look of admiration at one of the testers.

From the back, one rider looks about six feet tall, in his late-thirties, and overweight. Rolls of fat hang over the waistline of his jeans. He's riding a bike so he's moving, but, of course, not really moving because the wheels rest on a treadmill. All the Harley-Davidson advertisements in the lobby really emphasize that sense of the open road, an unfettered adult on the loose across the great American landscape.

Of course so many of us now drive cars and motorcycles that our highways have become sluggish with traffic. It's impossible to "fly" on the open road near any major metro area in the United States. And the workers themselves who put together the motorcycles live confined physical lives that have them moving, but not really moving in ways that would make their bodies strong and healthy.

Looking at the back of this American worker, I see all the things that have gone awry with our contract between our bodies and our jobs.

Once again, I am overcome with an urge to leave.

6

Action and Stillness in Nature

How Do Animals Achieve a Healthy Balance?

After focusing on movement for more than a year, I came across an article in the *New York Times* about sleep. On average humans shut down 7.7 hours a night, for reasons scientists can't explain, which puts us somewhere between the baboon (9.4) and the gray seal (6.2). Of course my teenage daughter often snoozes for ten hours or more on the weekends, which ranks right up there with the three-toed sloth.

So much of what we know about nature comes from dramatic TV documentaries that show cheetahs running sixty miles per hour in pursuit of dinner. In fact these endangered cats sleep at least fifteen hours a day and sometimes have to rest thirty minutes or more after they make a kill just to recover enough energy to eat. Stillness is just as much a part of life on Earth as action. Any time a creature moves it burns calories, which it must replace by finding more food; quest too far for too long without success and you die.

"There's a basic equation: habitat and food equals activity level," says John Gibbons, my red-headed, trim guide at the National Zoo in Washington, D.C., where I've come to learn more about where humans fall on nature's movement continuum.

"There's no need to chase a tree or stalk a bush," he adds, as we stand in front of the silverback in the lowland gorilla exhibit. The alpha male, which has a head the size of the tires on my Volvo, squats next to a pile of grass.

He looks incredibly muscular for a loafer, and I can't help but think that he would be roaming if he could. But throughout my tour, John warns me about anthropomorphizing the creatures behind the glass.

"People come up to me and say, 'Gosh, they should be able to move around a lot more.' But then I ask them: 'If you weren't here, where would you be?'" He pauses before he answers his own question. "Sitting on the couch in front of the TV."

Of course, even if I come to accept that the astounding specimen in front of me would be following a similar low-key physical routine in the wild, I still empathize with his lack of control. A detailed sign next to the glass enclosure explains that gorillas do not like direct eye contact. Visitors should approach the viewing area with downcast eyes and with their backs to the animals.

No one follows gorilla etiquette. We all stare boldly and with curiosity at the primates. During a separate trip I made to the zoo, a young boy shouted, "Whoa!" when he saw the silverback and ran up to slap the window, which made a thwacking sound. If we were in the wild, I can't imagine the silverback taking that sitting down.

At the cheetah enclosure, John points out the four one-year-old cubs and their mother. They lounge in a group, relishing the warmth of their collective body heat on a chilly January day. Large spools rest in the dirt throughout the yard. Zoo staffers thread a big rope through the spools then attach objects to the strand. When they yank the line things flip and twitch and the cheetahs start pouncing.

"It's like a lure course for a dog," John explains. "We have a physical enrichment program for nearly all the animals except maybe some of the fish. We even have an enrichment program for the octopus."

In the 1970s zoos in the United States became more interested in linking their work to conservation efforts and focused more on meeting the needs of each species not only on a dietary level but also on a physical, emotional, and social level.

"What does the cheetah need to maintain its cheetahness, if you will," is how John explained it.

In his book *The Human Zoo*, Desmond Morris, one-time curator of the London zoo, writes at length about the different needs of specialists versus opportunists. Specialists have only one thing they feel impelled to do, like an anteater needs ants or a panda needs bamboo. Opportunists, like wolves and primates (including humans), are jacks-of-all-trades and survive by taking advantage of a variety of environments.

"They evolved nervous symptoms that abhor inactivity," Morris writes, "that keep them constantly on the go."

If you cage opportunists, they often do weird things, like attack their offspring, develop stomach ulcers, mutilate themselves, and get fat, which, as Morris points out, is precisely the behavior patterns many human city dwellers sink into. The struggle for stimuli replaces the struggle for survival.

I mention Morris's book to John as we walk by the Mexican wolf, resplendent in her winter fur and lying quietly on the ridge about 100 feet away. John admires her coat—"so spectacular this time of year"—and falls silent.

The gray seal, which shares the human penchant for seven hours of sleep a day, lives right across from the wolf in a pool fringed with rocks. I think of the sleep chart as I watch "Silky" swim slowly from one ledge to another and imagine that this, then, is where a human would fall on the movement continuum at the zoo: not as frisky as the sea lion next door or as bored as the long-trekking wolf, but rather a sleeper on par with the gray seal.

"Gray seals eat sea urchins, which don't move, so their food source isn't too active," John says, in an effort to make, once again, the connection between food and physical-activity habits.

"If you take the whole wild kingdom—fish, insects—we're one of the less active species. But among mammals, we're probably mid-range. Of course, if you had asked this question 5,000 years ago, the answer would be very different because of what's happened to our food sources. Why hunt down food if you can get it to come to you [think farming and refrigerators]. So the answer is different now."

Clearly, given the high rate of diabetes, cancer, heart disease, and obesity among modern Americans, in this case "different" is not better.

Nature makes use of movement and stillness with remarkable precision and purpose. A peek at just a small sampling of the physical-activity patterns of some species reveals a world where the difference between life and death literally rests on respecting the balance between action and inaction.

I shall begin with hummingbirds because each summer I watch them at my feeder on the porch of a small cottage in New Hampshire, so I have heard firsthand the whirl of their passing and seen, through binoculars, their breasts vibrating with as many as 1,200 heartbeats per minute. They are one of the few wild species that still come into the viewfinder of my modern life.

Hovering flight is the most demanding form of locomotion in the animal kingdom, which explains why the hummingbird needs more energy than any other bird and must visit more than 1,000 flowers a day to survive. Most species stay in the rainforests of Central and South America, but the Ruby-throated hummingbirds I see migrate 2,500 miles (4,000 kilometers) between my New Hampshire feeder and South America every season. To pull this off they must fly 500 miles nonstop across the Gulf of Mexico. It takes four million wing beats to make the trip. If they don't double their body weight before the attempt, they drop like a stone no bigger than my thumb and drown.

Then there are the species that have perfected stillness: the praying mantis that imitates the life of a stick until prey comes within reach; the three-toed sloth that sleeps like a human teenager, but takes advantage of its super-slow lifestyle to grow a coat of blue-green algae on its fur during the rainy season, which helps camouflage it from predators.

The general rule of thumb in nature is that small, quick movers live short lives while methodical types live longer (a sloth can last as long as forty years in the treetops of South America while a frantically mating mayfly is lucky to live two days).

The most successful species, insects, took a huge leap forward on the evolutionary chain when they developed wings. Their greater mobility led them to a wider variety of food sources and improved their chances against predators. The shrew-like creature that many scientists believe was the common ancestor for all mammals today had a similar lucky break: its warm blood allowed it to remain active at all hours while the cold-blooded reptiles had to wait for the morning sun.

Every living creature is a mover and shaker according to the needs of the niche that it fills. Is it a pollinator of flowers (bees and my hummingbirds), a spreader of seeds (birds and squirrels), an opportunist with few predators and a wide range of food choices (wolves, humans, and other primates)? On every level, right down to the placement of its internal organs, a creature is born to move in certain ways.

Even plants move according to a carefully honed plan that evolved over generations. As biology professor and author Bernd Heinrich points out in his delightful book, *The Trees in My Forest*, the tilt of leaves to the sun, the growth of a central trunk in relation to spiraling branches, even the height of leaves from the ground are all part of an elaborate dance a plant engages in to find light, water, and minerals. A tree on the steppe of Africa may need to avoid giraffes so it grows a long, branchless trunk with leaves in bunches way above even the blue-tongued grazer's reach. A pine in Maine, however, must have its branches move in a spiral, layered pattern so the heavy winter snows can slough off harmlessly.

Charles Darwin was the first researcher to write about all of this in his book *The Power of Movement in Plants*. He noticed that "the habit of moving at certain periods is inherited both by plants and animals." His studies revealed some force other than light that encourages grasses to move and grow vertically. Later scientists learned that plants actually have hormones, just like animals, that have a major impact on plants' growth and movement patterns in relation to soil and light.

So the question for humans is how much can we fiddle with our inherent humanness, if you will, and still remain true to our movement mandate? Has our sedentary lifestyle already forced us across a line and the next step is to change ourselves on a biological level to better accommodate our new patterns?

Scientists are looking into it.

Bears, for example, can hibernate for months then emerge at full strength. Researchers have actually braved grizzly bear dens in winter to snag blood samples for a chemical tale that might answer why. Bears hibernate to avoid starvation (not the cold), but why do they accumulate huge amounts of vitamin C in their brains and spine? They don't urinate while hibernating, which would normally lead to a dangerous buildup of nitrogen. They dodge that bullet by converting the nitrogen into protein. The end result: no loss of muscle mass and no need to take a drink.

Astronauts, on the other hand, who travel in space for two weeks lose 3 to 13 percent of their bone and muscle mass; a paraplegic loses about 30 percent just six months after an accident. Can we learn from the bear how to program our bodies so they'll become better adapted to staying still? It's one thing to use such technology to help a person with paralyzed legs, but what about an overweight, couch-sitting, middle-aged man?

For now scientists are more interested in helping the truly needy, but just as hormone-replacement therapy spilled over into the mass marketplace, especially among body builders, bear juice could catch on mighty quick among Americans who want the sedentary lifestyle without all the nasty side effects. Want to watch five hours of television every day, eat steak and fries, and drink a six-pack of beer? Go ahead. Just be sure to take that pill so you can awake the next day at full strength and not a pound heavier!

It sounds creepy, but the human body may not be as far off the bear template as it first appears. In a 2005 issue of *Science* magazine, a group of scientists reported that they'd put mice into a hibernating state and then rejuvenated them with no adverse effects by gassing them with hydrogen sulfide, which reduced oxygen at the cellular level. The body temperature of the mice dropped from 98 to 58 degrees and their breathing fell from 120 to 10 breaths per minute. Basically they transformed the mice from warm-blooded to cold-blooded creatures. The authors think that humans have a latent ability to hibernate but don't harness it.

Of course hydrogen sulfide is highly toxic, and the experiment only worked with low, carefully administered amounts, but imagine if ambulance workers could put a person suffering from a heart attack into a hibernating state until they could reach the hospital. The whole idea of suspended animation has been around a long time, but the mouse experiment shows it may very well be in reach. It's not a huge leap of faith to assume that humans could enjoy *all* the benefits of hibernation.

As we come to the end of our tour at the zoo, John and I walk at a brisk clip. When I first met him, I assured him I had worn sensible shoes and would welcome an extended tour. General physical fitness has declined so much in the United States that someone like John can no longer assume that a middle-aged woman like myself can make the half-mile walk to the Ape House.

We started slowly, but by the time we reached the Mexican wolf, we picked up the pace. I began to sweat under my sweater. John started to look relaxed and invigorated. He said he welcomed any chance to get away from his desk, and he said this as though he were sharing a secret with a person who had the same "problem."

Last year he sold his car because he only lives a mile from the zoo.

"My friends sat me down and had this serious conversation with me. They wanted to be sure I really knew what I was doing and that I understood it was a really big decision. 'A mile is a long way,' they said."

At this point we're walking up a steep hill. The animals are behind us. This is my favorite part of the tour, just talking with another person, who not only cares about fitness, but also has thought about his own fitness patterns.

John tells me he works out at the gym regularly, but he also tries to include more casual exercise in his general day, like walking the mile to work. He understands the need for both approaches to movement in his life. I'm shocked. In all of my travels from Kansas to the Capital, he's the first person, besides Bill Sands at the Olympic Center, to verbalize this vital distinction. He knows what I know, I think to myself, and what I've only learned by doing the research for this book. For a moment I actually feel less lonely.

I see this same sense of simpatico occur between my daughter and her more active girlfriends. By middle school, most girls practically stop in their tracks and start spending their extra energy on trips to the mall or on computer games and TV shows at home. Someone who tries to stay active is ostracized as incredibly unhip. You simply do not play volleyball or build sand castles at the beach; you lounge on the towel in the sun for hours. You simply do not play tag or shoot hoops at recess; you sit under the tree, gossip, and watch the boys play football. If, on the off chance, my daughter actually bumps into a girl her age who wants to ski, sled, swim, or do anything physically active, an instant bond forms. "Ah, I finally found someone like me," her face says.

Which is precisely how I felt as I talked with John at the zoo; finally someone who understands.

But that means that movement patterns have become a major social marker among Americans. And here are the primary categories:

- Nearly 50 percent do no activity and watch hours of TV every day.
- Less than 5 percent exercise to extreme and often damage their bodies

(think ultra marathoners and Ironman competitors); this category has seen significant growth in the last five years.

◉ About 40 percent do some sort of moderate exercise every week, but that's counting light walks.

◉ An unknown percentage, but probably around 10 percent, work out pretty rigorously three or more times a week (a thirty-minute swim, for example) and also incorporate light exercise into the general flow of their day (walks of a mile or so or chores that involve going up and down stairs).

I have moved from the Ironman category to the final category, which healthcare professionals label "integrative exercise," which still leaves me with less than 10 percent of the American population to relate to on a physical level. For my daughter the percentage is probably even lower.

"Movement for leisure is a purely human thing," says John. "The idea, 'Let's go for a walk,' is an incredible human notion." But perhaps therein lies the problem. We've found a way to make physical activity a choice and to undo all of this damage we need to make it a lifestyle requirement again. John got rid of his car so now he *has* to walk to work.

We finish our walk at the visitors' center, shake hands, and John departs. On my way out, I pause at the cheetah yard. One thing I learned about nature's movement continuum at the zoo is that stillness plays a much larger role in the wild than I thought. Most species spend most of their lives in a quiet state. Visitors are lucky if they see the cheetahs, the fastest mammal on the earth, do anything but lounge. Perhaps the fact that Americans sit in front of a TV instead of by a pile of savannah grass is not that big a deal.

But then I recall the expression on John's face when he looked down at my shoes. Relief. I could walk a mile with him.

No, I decide, if a fellow American can't be certain that a woman in her prime can walk a mile in her shoes then we've carried the stillness thing too far.

7

Action and Stillness in Humans

Can Americans Achieve a Healthy Balance?

I return to the National Zoo in springtime, when flower petals speckle the asphalt and sidewalk. This time instead of watching the animals, I want to talk with and observe people who live around the zoo, which is one of the most eclectic neighborhoods in the Capital area, with large communities of Hispanic immigrants, African Americans, young professionals, and wealthy whites. In general the sidewalks run wide, the blocks have a rich blend of shops, and it's about as walkable an area as anyone will find in the United States. Whatever I see here with regard to healthy physical activity patterns will be about as good as it gets.

I begin at the zoo gate, which faces Connecticut Avenue, and turn left toward the Calvert Street Bridge. I keep walking until I hit the 3000 block of 16th Street, the land of the sensible shoes. I spend two hours watching as hundreds of people walk by, all of them wearing either sneakers or some other low-heeled shoe. The women, mostly Hispanic or African American, usually pull a small cart packed with groceries. The men walk, too, though they also zip by on bicycles, without helmets, toe clips, lights, reflecting vests, or any of the other safety equipment that's common in more affluent neighborhoods. Fewer people own a car in this area, known as Ward 1 down at city hall, than any other area in D.C.

There are long lines at the bus stop, and most of the cars pass through. Only two drivers try to park during the two hours I sit there in the late afternoon. The official head count for Latinos in Washington is about 9 percent of the population, but the city's own Office of Latino Affairs admits a huge "undercount" and estimates the real number is closer to 15 percent and growing at a much faster rate than any other segment of the population. The majority came here from El Salvador, and more than half of them settle in this one neighborhood.

I've arranged to have a translator meet me, a health professional named Matilde Palmer, who grew up in the Dominican Republic, where she worked as a general physician before she married an American then settled in Bethesda, Maryland, to raise her two boys. We meet at the Family Place, a nonprofit organization that helps young Latina women with children under age five adjust to life in the U.S.

The tight, three-story townhouse has peeling green paint on the front porch and a modest sign. Inside it's all blue and white, tidy and bright. Young women bustle up and down the stairs with babies on their hips or toddlers in front. Matilde herself is petite and stylishly accessorized with designer angular glasses, a leather jacket, and jewelry.

The women speak in rapid-fire, animated Spanish that I cannot follow, though it's clear that they are overjoyed to see Matilde and even seem a bit in awe of her. She runs parenting classes at the clinic and knows the women well.

All of them but one have long, thick brown hair, expressive eyes, large earrings, simple but tight-fitting clothing, and quick smiles. They eat vegetables and rice provided by the center while we sit and talk. Matilde tells them that I am interested in their physical activity habits now that they live in the United States and how those habits differ from what they used to do in their native countries.

I quickly learn the basics: several of them are from El Salvador and one is from Guatemala. They help at a dry cleaners, work as a janitor at a school, and as a maid. They must always walk or take the bus to their jobs.

They miss their homelands and recall childhoods packed with manual labor.

"I brought wood to help my mother with her cooking fire."

"I worked in the store from age five."

"I cleaned the wheat."

The woman who worked the fields has cropped hair and a broad face. She's from Guatemala and remembers that it "was hard work, but I miss being outdoors with a group and on the move."

The women eat quietly after she says this. One of them quickly adds that she feels very fortunate to have a good job here and likes her work here too. Then all is silent again, and only the young boy on one mother's knee makes noise.

All of them must get to work so they leave their children with the center and head off, a chattering group heading out to the bus.

It's clear that none of these women has the money or time to take anything like an exercise class, and while they certainly have physically demanding jobs, all of them are overweight. They've incorporated walking and lots of physical activity into their daily lives but it's not working for them in terms of their overall health because the American diet undermines many of those gains.

Matilde agrees and explains, "In my country and their countries, you did not have the privilege of going to a restaurant. But then people come here and they see McDonalds and are so excited that they can take their family to a restaurant. But it's not a real restaurant, you know what I mean, and it's bad for them, but they don't know that. All they know is that they can afford it."

We head over to a couch in a side room. The light from the window catches Matilde's face—she has lovely high cheeks and engaged eyes. She's clearly thought long and hard about the health issues faced by immigrants and deals with them at her clinic and at the Family Place everyday.

"Obesity is the biggest health complication," she says. "What they all need is knowledge."

But Matilde's own story shows that "knowledge" alone, in terms of educational programs and information, will never be enough. She recalls a childhood in the Dominican Republic where they walked everywhere, climbed trees well into their teens, and raced around the sugarcane fields sucking on the cane. They played pick up games of baseball and stayed outside until sunset.

Her own sons have a much better standard of living, but then she sees them "engaged in so much electronics and TV, and I ask them to go outside for one hour and they think it's so much. And the competitive sports got them discouraged so they don't want to go anymore."

Her homeland continues to struggle economically, and she knows this is a better place for them, but she feels the loss of their physical life and the health and social consequences of that loss. What she left wasn't right, especially for the people working the sugarcane fields, but what she found isn't right either.

We talk of bags of potato chips for 99 cents and $2 mangos, which pretty much sums up why so many immigrants wind up mimicking American eating patterns; fresh produce is simply way too expensive here. As we walk out of the Family Place together, I realize that what I've learned by coming down in person to the streets just confirms what I've been reading about for years: immigrants and other disadvantaged Americans struggle more than any other group with poor diet, lack of consistent exercise, and the resulting health consequences.

The next day I return to the National Zoo entrance again, but this time I take my car and turn right up Connecticut Avenue toward Cleveland Park, also known as Ward 3. I want to navigate deep up the avenue and have limited time so I drive. I pass metro stops, grocery stores like Magruder's—packed with produce and organic foods—bikers decked out in all sorts of gear, lots of walkers, but women in heels too. Here, most people have a college degree. Here, most people have cars and twice as much money as the people in Ward 1.

I've lined up some interviews with several young, white, single professionals who live in the apartments that face the avenue. I pass a Gold's Gym just before their block, which is packed with dozens of white, young professional-types on stationary bikes and treadmills with their backs to each other but facing the street. The backlight from the exercise room highlights each of them as dusk closes in outside. I know it's fantastic that they are moving, that they have the time and money to get in there and sweat, but it's a spectacular spring evening outside and they all look so disconnected from each other and the outdoors. This is not a group spontaneously moving through their day, but, as far as I can tell, this is the best default posture that Americans have found—the scheduled, measured, regimented workout.

I admit that I entered the elevator of the apartment building brimming with assumptions about the twentysomething recent college graduates I was about to meet. I figured they took full advantage of the great food markets in the neighborhood, the simple walk to the Metro, and the exercise classes offered at places like Gold's Gym. I assumed their world was packed with healthy choices and any struggles they might have to stay physically active and to sustain a healthy diet were self-created issues.

Rachel Winch puts me in my place immediately. She's young, white, single, new to Washington by way of California and Connecticut, working for a nonprofit, living on a tight budget, and frustrated by the choices that American grocery stores and America's landscape hand her.

"I am not trying to say I am in the same situation as the Latina women you interviewed, but I am down to a piece of fresh fruit a day and have been eating canned fruit. I have to go to multiple stores to avoid substituting crap for good food. My point here," she says, as she sits on the edge of a worn couch, "is that even those of us for whom all of this is central to our lives, who care deeply about physical activity and nutrition, the conditions are stacked against us."

In California, it was easier on all levels, she confides. She could find affordable fresh produce and found safe bicycle lanes everywhere.

"Of course, D.C. isn't as bad as, say, Alabama," where riding her bike on any road was usually a life-threatening experience because there were no shoulders and drivers weren't used to sharing the road.

Her roommate, Taylor Godfrey, also young, white, single, and working on Capitol Hill, shies away from biking, but does walk whenever he can, especially to the Metro. "For me, it's about a sense of accomplishment. I like to be able to say at the end of the day I have done XYZ," a mindset the stationary bikers back at Gold's Gym probably share. But then Taylor looks away for a moment, his classic Scottish profile caught in the kitchen light, and confides that he often comes home way too spent to even try an exercise routine on a machine. Up on the Hill, he says, the young staffers at least try to do some activity, but the old-timers, well, no.

They both kept physical activity diaries for me. Taylor walked a lot and then uncorked a five-mile run after not running for almost ten days; a feat usually left best to the young. Rachel is clearly more deliberate about her physical activity choices and walks, bikes, dances, does yoga, and takes stairs. Lots and lots of stairs. She became really deliberate about it after reading *Prescription for a Healthy Nation*, by Tom Farley and Deborah Cohen, which explores how city planning and our physical environment shape and limit our exercise options.

Of course, when Rachel made up her mind to boycott elevators, she didn't think about how spooky and deserted most stairwells are or how difficult it can be to find the doors to stairwells in most buildings with elevators. All of these factors just made her more determined because it further proved her point and the book authors' point that the way we design the physical structures in our lives forces us into more sedentary habits.

"We are *all* impacted by structures that limit physical activity," she says, with a huge emphasis on *all*. "And it doesn't just impact us physically. It's the mental space too." Yes, I think getting caught in a stairwell is a suffocating experience and so is getting caught at a desk all day at work. Your body wants to move and your mind wants to breathe.

I think about the wolf back at the zoo; another opportunist limited by his environment and desperately seeking stimulation.

When I ask both Taylor and Rachel what sort of physical life they would like to have in a perfect world, they both list huge amounts of activity.

"I could easily see myself running three to four miles a day and walking another four to five," says Taylor.

"What my body wants," Rachel pauses, then says with a big smile, "to bike thirty miles a day and walk five. Right now I bike about fifteen miles a day and walk two or three most days and I still feel a little antsy."

Taylor stands, sipping water. Rachel stands and sits then stands again throughout our conversation. They both seem as unnaturally contained as the Gold Gym regulars.

"I want to live a life where exercise becomes hard to quantify," Rachel adds. "It just is."

This young woman, still pressing the boundaries of what she wants her professional and personal life to be, has just captured the essence of what I want to see in terms of physical activity in American culture.

It just is.

The people in Ward 1 long for it. The people in Ward 3 long for it. No matter what an individual's economic or ethnic background, most Americans want and need a more spontaneous amount of physical activity in their lives, and they can't simply will their way through the obstacles.

I take Rachel's advice and read *Prescription for a Healthy Nation,* which points out that from 1890 to 1990 only 15 percent of the huge increase in life expectancy could be attributable to medical care, such as vaccines or improvements in surgical procedures. Instead, it was *preventive* care, including cleaning up the drinking water and sewage disposal, that brought about the most health benefits. Half of all deaths in the United States today are caused by individual human behavior, such as poor diet or lack of exercise, and yet as a nation we spend less than three-tenths of 1 percent of healthcare dollars on preventive measures.

Simply spreading the gospel of a healthier diet and physical activity three times a week for thirty minutes has resulted in some progress, but the fact remains that about half of the population continues to pursue very unhealthy eating and physical-activity patterns. In one study that Farley and Cohen cite, a group of high school teens in Baltimore were bombarded with messages about the horrors of cigarette smoking. The end result: they had a much darker view of smoking as a habit, but did not actually alter their own behavior as smokers very much because it was so central to their social lives.

I think back to Matilde's McDonald's story. Even if she tells many of the newly arrived immigrants that the fatty burgers and greasy fries are horrible for their health, they would go, because others go, because it's wonderful to go "out" for a meal because the food tastes so different from what they fix at home. Even if I tell my teenage daughter she should exercise five times a week, if she must do it alone, or squeeze it into a schedule packed with theater and studying, it won't happen.

"Because our nation's leading killers are behaviors like smoking, high calorie diets, sedentary behavior and drinking, the fight that really matters," the authors of *Prescription for a Healthy Nation* conclude, "are the ones over the *design* of our world as it shapes our behaviors."

"The only way the majority of Americans are going to get moving is if activity is part of their daily routines. It has to be as unavoidable as an encounter with a vending machine is now."

After talking with people in Washington and spending more time observing in the neighborhoods around the National Zoo, I believe the linchpin is the underlying assumption that exercise is something that we "go" to or "choose" to do. This attitude evolved by the turn-of-the-twentieth century as more people worked jobs that involved very little physical activity and had to turn to biking or long strolls, for example, in their leisure time to get moving.

But the fact remains that until at least 1920, at least half of Americans were still working on farms, and the rise of the desk culture has only been firmly entrenched among the majority for about sixty to seventy years. If we go back to incorporating movement throughout our days, we would be returning to the norm, not leaving it.

By 1960 only a quarter of Americans did regular exercise. That figure jumped up to about 50 percent by 1980, a leap that everyone rightly hailed as a major accomplishment. Fueled by trends set in motion by fitness gurus like muscle man Jack LaLanne (1960s), runner Frank Shorter (who won the marathon at the 1972 Olympics), and Jane Fonda fitness tapes and copycats (1980s), Americans started to get into their bodies. A 1981 *Time* magazine cover story, "America Shapes Up," spent ten pages on the new obsession with youthfulness and the money pouring into companies like Nike, but just one page on the health benefits of the new habits. The prevailing view for many, including the famous Chicago newspaperman Studs Terkel: "working on your body is narcissistic."

By the late 1990s the health benefits of just about any form of exercise had become abundantly clear and communicated to the general population. In 1998, *The Futurist* magazine ran an article that captured the shift in attitudes. More people worked out to "maintain health and vitality rather than appearance." The top forms of exercise: weights, stationary bikes, treadmills, walking outside, and running.

Today, the connection between moving and overall health is beyond dispute and embraced as a given by the American public. In just forty years, even though just half of us exercise as often as we should, almost all of us have undergone a major shift in attitude and accept that moving should be part of our daily lives. Now to make that happen in the physical landscapes that we live in, and in the work schedules most of us keep, is a different challenge, but the mental topsoil has been laid.

In 2008 the American College of Sports Medicine did a global poll of 10,000 people on what they felt was most important in fitness today. The top-ten list:

◎　　Educated and experienced fitness professionals
◎　　Exercise programs for children fighting obesity

◎   Personal trainer

◎   Strength trainer

◎   Core training

◎   Special fitness program for older adults

◎   Pilates

◎   Functional fitness

◎   Swiss ball

◎   Yoga

Now this is a list firmly rooted in "going" to exercise; there's no call for systemic changes. But the fact yoga made the top ten is encouraging, since it's a form of exercise that shirks competition and doesn't focus on building showy muscles, but celebrates tone, balance, an aligned body, good breathing techniques, and mental discipline. According to a Roper poll commissioned by *Yoga Journal*, eleven million Americans do yoga occasionally and six million do it regularly. People have practiced this Indian import for an estimated 3,000 years, but it didn't really take root in the U.S. until the 1960s. Back then it was often mocked as the exercise of choice for flighty hippies, but with less narcissistic attitudes toward fitness taking hold, mind/body routines like yoga have found a more universal acceptance.

Whenever people hear about what I'm working on for this book, they always suggest I try yoga. My back surgery made it almost impossible for me to hold most of the positions, so I have avoided an organized class and just do some of the stretches and breathing exercises on a weekly basis. Tai Chi, a Chinese form of exercise that is part martial arts and part meditation in motion, seemed more approachable so I enrolled at a local center.

Of course, I was still "going" to exercise, but I was hoping that what I learned there would make me more mindful of my body, balance, breathing, and focus *all day*. It would be exercise that would serve as a root for an overall attitude toward movement. It was the tulip bulb in the proverbial mental topsoil I mentioned earlier.

Tai Chi developed in China more than 2,000 years ago as a self-defense strategy. The folklore backdrop: a Taoist monk marveled at how a snake avoided the bird's thrusting beak and actually managed to use the bird's force against it. Tai Chi evolved to include more than 100 separate movements and postures.

An expert can execute each sequence in a slow but flawlessly flowing manner. The Chinese reorganized the number of postures several times, including a reduction to twenty-four core forms in 1956. The slowness is supposed to encourage a person to be fully in the moment even as he or she moves with lightness and balance.

I decided my last man-in-the-street interviews would be in a Tai Chi class, where people choose to attend but also embrace a philosophy of movement that's meant to carry over into their daily lives. The group that gathers around the instructor is white, middle aged, in varying states of fitness, and all women. The instructor herself is petite with long brown hair, no make-up and in loose cotton trousers. I try to chat a bit with the others about why they are here, but they dodge the conversation and clearly want to start.

The instructor greets us with her hands: a flat palm on top of a fist. The tight violence of the lower hand reminds me that this is also a form of martial arts and each stance is somewhat combative; the hand movements are like "knives." (The instructor's word, not mine.) As a former basketball player, I enjoy the fact I am in a low crouch and must pivot on the balls of my feet, but I balk at the slow, deliberate nature of the movements. I shift my weight onto my back hip, slowly swing a foot forward, and try to unravel my long arms the way she unravels hers. I become very mindful of my unusually large wingspan and long fingers. I realize I am looking in a mirror of sorts and must move in the opposite direction of the instructor because she is facing us. I find this confusing and repeatedly must start again.

Indeed, while I'm clearly the most athletic person in the room, I am most certainly not the most comfortable. The others seem less jittery and more accepting of the methodical pace and deliberate sequencing. I want to move freely, as though taking a jump shot in one quick motion. My frayed lower disks strain to hold one position for long, and my damaged left ankle does not like carrying my full body weight. My competitive, intense nature works against me here. To succeed, I must feel that it's less about performance and more about centering myself in relation to the floor, my spine, and my surgically repaired back. I must breathe through my nose and out through my mouth.

To make it work, I must accept that it's about flow. I cannot choose to make that happen; it must move through me naturally like a wave.

8

A Tour Through Sixty Years of Advice

Matilde, Rachel, and Taylor touched upon many things that keep them and people they know from being more physically active, but they live in a small area—diverse, densely populated, and very walkable—but still just one patch in a big nation. Are their complaints—lack of time, no easy access, fear of public spaces—the complaints of the masses?

I decide to look through the huge databases of federal agencies that work to get Americans moving. The titles, programs, subprograms, and contact information listed on federal home pages alone could fill a small phone book. Like some perky cyberspace commercial, the upbeat names show when I Google "Physical Activity AND Americans": Steps for a Healthier U.S., Action for Healthy Kids, Healthy People 2010, Hearts and Parks, EPA Smart Growth, the Nutrition and Physical Activity Program to Prevent Obesity and Other Chronic Diseases. And on it goes.

If I leap to the nonprofit sector, the list expands exponentially: Rails and Trails, YMCA Wellness Program, National Center for Minority Health, American Heart Association, National Association of Sport and Physical Education, American College of Sports Medicine . . .

Amid all the wellness chatter, most of it well-meaning, I found a rare flash of bluntness on the Surgeon General's site, which issued an official statement of bafflement: "Despite common knowledge that exercise is helpful, more than 60 percent of American adults are not regularly active and 25 percent of the adult population are not active at all." In government speak that's essentially asking, "What gives?" The information is definitely getting out there and hundreds of thousands of medical and fitness professionals devote their careers to the problem; but, on the whole, the American population remains dangerously, resolutely immobile.

Scientists predict that the collective inertia of my own baby-boomer generation will be directly responsible for as much as $32.4 *billion* in health-care costs by 2020, as we sit and sag our way to retirement. Clearly there are a lot of people out there who simply don't care; but there are also a lot of people out there like Matilde, Rachel, and Taylor who do and still struggle. I stop my web journey to take the "Barriers to Being Active Quiz" on the Centers for Disease Control and Prevention (CDC) website. "What keeps you from being more active?" it bluntly asks.

"Question One: How likely are you to say:

1. My day is so busy now, I just don't think I can make time to include physical activity in my regular schedule."
    Am I   "Very Likely" (3), "Somewhat Likely" (2), "Somewhat Unlikely (1), or "Very Unlikely" (0) to give this answer?

I think of how often I don't walk because I don't feel I have the time and circle "Somewhat Likely" for two points. The quiz has a total of twenty-one declarative statements, such as "I really can't see learning a new sport at my age." I circle "Very Unlikely" for zero points on that one. Or "None of my family members or friends like to do anything active, so I don't have a chance to exercise." I know my teenage daughter (thinking of her fellow teens) would circle "Very Likely" for three points on that one, but I say "no" and nail zero.

As I move my way down the page, marking two points here and zero there, I already see my own pattern: lack of time.

At the end of the quiz, the CDC has seven basic categories: lack of time, social influence, lack of energy, lack of will power, fear of injury, lack of skill, and lack of resources. I plug the appropriate numbers into each of the seven lines and come up with a six under "Lack of Time." Any score over five "shows that this is an important barrier for you to overcome."

"Lack of energy" comes in a distant second for me, but I barely register even a one in the other five categories.

I step back from my standup desk and look at the list of seven formulas on my computer screen. The words *fear* and *lack* leap out at me: so my random sweep through the D.C. neighborhoods proved spot on. What's really keeping Americans in their seats? Well, based on this primitive quiz, a lack of discipline, skewed priorities, insecurity, a lack of access to safe recreational areas, and money.

I scroll down the page and read the CDC's suggestions on how to conquer *fear* and *lack*, but their sampler sounds all too familiar, like an old commercial jingle.

- Identify at least three thirty-minute time slots you could use for physical activity.
- Explain your interest in physical activity to friends and family Ask them to support your efforts.
- Plan ahead.
- Join an exercise class or group.
- Encourage exercise facilities to provide childcare services.

Just like the relentlessly optimistic names of all the wellness programs I found on the Internet, this list glides like sugared water through my mind. Empty calories and predictable solutions we've all heard so many times before.

When I skip to the USDA home page, I find other pat suggestions on how to get moving: use stairs, walk, garden. Of course all of these are splendid things, and I do all three deliberately as part of my effort to increase the activity quotient of my average day, but none of these answers gets at the deeper reasons why Americans aren't moving, and why even a stair-climbing guru like Rachel Winch feels caged in by the physical (and dietary) constraints imposed on her by American culture.

While navigating the U.S. Department of Agriculture (USDA) site, which includes a lot of pages on physical-activity programs for kids, I come across something that reflects a damaging philosophical shift that takes place between the late childhood years and adulthood. While the USDA advises adults to try gardening and walking, it urges kids to be "spontaneously active." We ALL need to be spontaneously active but that category disappears on the adult pages.

I also noticed that all of the government sites use passive voice, which means the verbs have no clear subjects. That allows the CDC, Health and Human Services (HHS), the USDA, and any other federal program to let the individual off the hook. The rise in weight "has been" dramatic. The decline in physical activity "has been" steady. Precisely who has gained the weight and caused the decline is rarely stated outright. Some sites might mention the impact of sprawl on people's walking patterns, but rarely call for Americans to accept blame for their own eating and physical habits. Even nonprofits in the private sector remain reticent to demand any personal accountability for the nation's sedentary multitudes. Whenever I talk with wellness professionals, they always balk when I ask them if they think it's odd that the executive director of a major public health organization is sixty pounds overweight or that parents allow their kids to go to school with soda and prepackaged junk food high in fat, salt, and sugar.

"Maybe he has a thyroid problem," they say about the director.

Another common refrain: "The kids will just buy the same soda from the vending machines at school so the parents might as well accept it."

They could be right on both counts, of course, but I like to remain optimistic and believe that they are wrong. I like to believe that at least two-thirds of the nation's lifestyle problems could be remedied if the federal government, local programs, schools, employers, and parents demanded more personal accountability in America, and if those same organizations and people pushed for major systemic changes that made it much easier for the average citizen to embrace a more spontaneous approach to exercise.

After my tour through the various federal government websites, I decide to pen my own quiz.

Answer each question with one of the following: Very Likely (3), Somewhat Likely (2), Somewhat Unlikely (1), Very Unlikely (0).

"How likely are you to say:

1. I have the right to move on a regular basis, both at work and where I live, and the government has an obligation to support and sustain that right.

2.   If I am denied the right, I feel spiritually and physically depleted, which makes such restrictions a violation of my constitutional "right to happiness."
3.   I live in a society full of choices and temptations, but ultimately I am responsible for my own diet and exercise regimen.

I take my own quiz and circle "Very Likely" for statements 1 and 2, but hesitate at 3 and decide to circle "Somewhat Likely" instead. I created stacked questions for a quiz that mirrors my own prejudices, and I still can't answer "Very Likely" to all three items! I can think of innumerable times when I wanted to walk or bike but couldn't because of time constraints or a lack of access to safe trails or safe bike lanes on the primary roads.

As my interviews at the Family Place proved, in the poorest urban areas, where the levels of physical activity are especially low, people have to worry about not only finding time, but also safe and tidy public spaces. Study after study has shown that if people have relatively easy access to bike trails, safe walking paths, and clean parks, they will increase their general activity levels by 25 percent.

So while public and private health programs do a lousy job holding Americans accountable for their unresponsiveness to our nation's activity crisis, the fact remains that many citizens are not slothful because they want to be. So many other elements come into play, including access, safety, control over their schedules, and money.

The CDC has done a solid job pinning down precisely *which* Americans are turning a deaf ear. Some of their conclusions:

◎   Widows and women in general are less active.
◎   Hispanics and African Americans are less active.
◎   The poor are less active.
◎   The less educated are less active.
◎   A lack of time is the primary reason why most Americans feel they can't be more active.

As Juliet Schor makes clear in her book, *The Overworked American,* the economy and society demand too much of most adults, especially single mothers and minorities living on the edge. The average person has just sixteen hours of leisure a week (that counts domestic chores and job-hours as "work"), which reflects a continual decline in leisure time in the United States since World War II. Working women with kids (note women on the top of the CDC's list of physically inactive people) are especially hard hit and often put in as much as eighty hours of domestic and job-related work each week.

"Every study I have seen on the topic," writes Schor, "has found that workers lack free choice of hours."

As a writer and college professor, I have tremendous control over my schedule and yet "lack of time" remains a major obstacle even for me when it comes to getting the activity I want in my day. How is a single Hispanic mother with two jobs and three kids supposed to cope with the problem? The consequences of her lousy diet and lack of exercise are huge—Hispanics are especially susceptible to diabetes—but so are the end results if she doesn't bring home those paychecks. It's easier to see and feel the impact of no money, so obviously that's where she devotes most of her energies.

The end result: most Americans come home so spent that they gravitate to "low energy" recreation for their "down" time, which translates into watching television, playing computer games, and other sedentary activities. People who grow up in sync with their bodies, and the deeply therapeutic and energizing aspects of even moderate exercise, are more apt to continue to make time for physical activity no matter how busy they get as adults. For others, exercise just becomes another chore, a thing to "master" like an obligation at work, which makes it as mentally taxing as cleaning the house. Finding ways to sustain the joy of movement that "spontaneous activity" implies as Americans move from their teen years to adulthood is as essential to the long-term success of any wellness program as improving access and the safety of public spaces. The federal government and nonprofit groups have failed miserably at addressing these kinds of emotional issues that lie at the heart of the physical-activity crisis.

Fortunately physical changes in the environment can and have convinced people to alter their activity habits. How inspiring to know that simply having more accessible bike lanes on major roads can increase ridership 25 percent. While roaming on my web tour, I came across the American Public Health

Association's home page. The APHA helps pull together organizations from across the country who participate in Public Health Week, a federally sponsored "event" that runs every April, which Bill Clinton signed into existence in 1995. The year I went, the theme just so happened to be "Designing Healthy Communities." I arranged to sit in the meeting as they discussed their plans for Public Health Week with program managers and wellness directors from across the country.

I admit I drove to the APHA office building in the Chinatown section of Washington, D.C., instead of taking the metro and walking. I had chores to do and a class across town to teach, which is just the sort of "excuse" most women usually give when it comes to adding walking instead of car travel to their day. Maybe personal responsibility is overrated and only accounts for, well, 50 percent of the problem? I laugh at how easily I let myself off the hook.

I settle into my seat in a room with about fifty other people. Most of them are managers of fitness-related programs for YMCA, HHS, CDC, EPA, and many of the other organizations I came across during my tour on the Internet. The two women in charge of running things spend a lot of time talking about tool kits, public relations packets, and media outlets. I realize after about an hour that they have little more to work with than words.

As Tom Farley and Deborah Cohen made clear in *Prescription for a Healthy Nation*, preventive care has taken a backseat to medical care in the United States since the early twentieth century, but to see the consequences at work right in front of me is unnerving. The *marketing* budget of the American Medical Association, which represents doctors, is bigger than the entire budget of the APHA. So the people in the room with me are left with enough resources to pull off something like a Public Health Week, when what we really need is substantial programming for a monster National Public Health Crisis Decade.

After everyone disperses, I ask the two women in charge if they knew about the CDC quiz, since they want to make their own quiz to hand out in tool kits. No, they have not. I point out how it's all about *fear* and *lack*, and that Americans must demand changes in their physical environment if they ever hope to really address these two key problems. They agree, but also make it clear that with their current budget and staff, the best the APHA can do is serve as a clearinghouse for information among all sorts of organizations that might not normally talk to each other.

Frustrated, I grill a trim middle-aged man who happened to sit next to me in the meeting. He has a short-cropped beard and the demeanor of a professor who bikes to class. It turns out Keith Laughlin directs the Rails and Trails program, an organization that works to convert old railroad lines into bike trails across the country. Now here is someone working on the ground level for real change on infrastructure that has proven to increase physical activity among Americans.

He admits they all "talk a language that only each of us understands." He also acknowledges that a one- or two-day event in April is hardly what the nation needs, though even that Band-Aid is better than nothing.

"I'm not sure how to measure 'success' stories," he says, staring thoughtfully in front of him instead of at me. "At least they're trying to get the word out."

Before he came to Rails and Trails, Keith worked for a time as a speechwriter for former Democratic presidential candidate Al Gore, who at least had fitness and the environment on his radar screen. But as the election gained steam, it became clear that physical activity and access to safe, clean public spaces was what policy wonks called a "mommy" issue, Keith said, a rather sexist way of saying it was viewed as a local issue. Things like Iraq were "daddy" issues and made it easier for the candidate to look presidential. So even for a candidate who cared and had a speechwriter really passionate about these issues, it felt difficult, even impossible, to place fitness and urban planning on the national agenda. Of course if they tallied the cost and fatalities caused by Americans' horrible lifestyle habits, they'd find the numbers probably far outweigh the deaths and expense of the Iraq war over the long haul. The key is all in the spin.

One the first things John F. Kennedy did when he became president was hold a conference on fitness. He formed the President's Council on Physical Fitness and Sports. I remember as a middle school girl in the 1970s, years after JFK's assassination, trying to earn a perfect score on all parts of the Presidential Fitness Test, including the 800-yard-run, the shuttle run, and, the bane of my existence, the touch-your-toes flexibility test. I know the gym teacher at my daughter's former middle school puts the kids through a similar series of tasks, though measured in meters now, for some sort of Presidential certificate. One president, one program, and forty years later schoolyards across the country still feel the impact.

The other side of this tale, of course, is that the federal government has aggressively spread the news about the need for more physical movement in people's daily lives since the Eisenhower administration, and yet year-after-year about 60 percent of Americans fail to meet the federal government's modest recommendations. The same number—the infamous 60 percent—that the Surgeon General's report pointed to with frustration and bafflement hasn't changed a bit for decades.

America has developed a Sedentary Majority.

How can any organization, never mind the understaffed, under-funded AHPA, move the intractable masses? I began fishing around for sample success stories that might bring some positive ideas to the table and came across a perfect fit: the anti-smoking campaigns. It's hard to fathom today that 67 percent of adult men in the United States smoked in the 1940s. (Women's cigarette use peaked in the 1960s, when 44 percent lit up regularly.) Today 20 percent of both sexes over age twenty-five smoke, which is still remarkably high given the hard and horrible facts about the consequences of using tobacco, but that's still an astounding drop. On a nationwide scale, people of every income level, race, sex, and educational level stopped smoking.

Certainly personal resolve, educational programs at schools, and public service announcements on television played a role, but so did changes in the environment, including aggressive laws that banned smoking in many public spaces. The government severely curtailed smokers' choices. Private and public individuals altered access, exerted huge social pressure, and banned smoking outright in key areas (no more lighting up in the airplane). A sound wave of political and personal will swept through American culture and with it changes that really improved people's lives.

As a nonsmoker and asthmatic, I have trouble relating to the difficulties of giving up something as nasty as cigarettes, but I *can* look at my own experience with the seatbelt in my car, which is another area where Americans underwent a collective change in their habits to save lives.

In 1968 the federal government passed a law requiring all new cars to have seatbelts. Despite this aggressive move, only 10 to 15 percent of Americans bothered to use them. I know when I got my license in the late 1970s, I was one of those young drivers who felt confined by the belt. I ignored all the educational programming (and nasty accident pictures) in my Driver's Education classes. Somewhere in the back of my teenage mind I knew I had a 55 percent greater risk of severe injury in a frontal crash without a seatbelt on, but it was just an abstract statistic.

Then individual states began passing mandatory seatbelt laws, including Connecticut, where I was living when a policeman pulled me over for my first speeding ticket. I remember rushing to snap in the seatbelt as the officer approached my car. He nailed me for speeding but didn't tag on the much heftier seatbelt violation. Still, after that incident, I began locking in. In my case money proved a bigger incentive than fear.

At this point every state, except New Hampshire (Live Seat Belt Free and Die), has a mandatory seatbelt use law, and the overall use rate has jumped from 10 percent to 75 percent. Americans are still behind other Northern European countries and Canada, where 90 to 95 percent of people wear a seatbelt, but the story is still a success story.

Millions of people altered their behavior for the sake of safety. They did it for lots of reasons, including because they became better educated about the consequences, but in the end, it was the collective social pressure that did the trick. Policemen rarely enforce seatbelt laws, but most of us click the lock on the belt anyway. The nonbelt user is no longer considered cool, just stupid and a menace. Four percent of drivers still belong to the hard-core "I'll-never-wear-a-seatbelt" club, and they account for 60 percent of the severe crashes. Unbelted drivers also have 50 percent higher hospital bills when they are in an accident than belted drivers.

Overweight, sedentary Americans have a lot in common with these derelict drivers: they drive up healthcare costs for everyone and lower their own life expectancy. The government needs to apply the "seat-belt fix" and make it easier for these people to make healthier choices on a daily basis.

Today all cars bleep drivers with a high-pitched, eight-second tone if people try to drive off without wearing their seatbelt. There's no way to bleep a person who spends too long on the couch or at the computer (not yet anyway), but the power of social pressure is considerable. These success stories convince me that Americans can make fundamental shifts in their behavior. Why can't federal, state, and local governments and the private sector come up with revolutionary programs and laws that get Americans moving again that rival or even exceed the anti-smoking and seatbelt campaigns? To do it they must build political will, tap into each citizen's personal resolve, enforce laws that help people add movement to their daily lives no matter where they work or live, and rethink urban and suburban planning in America so our built environments make it much easier for a larger percentage of the population to step outside their door and walk down the block. If the federal government can ban smoking on airplanes, it can ban housing developments that practically require residents to travel everywhere by car.

After the APHA meeting and my tour through the government websites, I was ready to hit the road again. My target this time: San Diego, headquarters of the Active Living Research Foundation, an organization devoted to finding ways to get Americans moving again. They were about to hold their annual conference, and I made up my mind to be there. After nearly two years of researching and writing about the human body and past patterns of movement, I wanted to know what sort of solutions the nation's top scientists and wellness program directors were coming up with for the twenty-first century. There'd be hundreds of professionals in San Diego talking about everything from stair use in buildings to encouraging free play among kids in public parks. With a budget in the $90 million range, ALR has the cash, the experts, and the agenda I was looking for.

9

Seeking Solutions in the Twenty-First Century

I look out the window at Reagan National Airport in Washington, D.C., as I prepare to board an American West airplane headed for San Diego, and deep emotions wet my eyes. I stare at a planet just above the rising morning light and realize that after six years of rehabilitating my broken body, I am finally able to sit for five hours in an airplane seat without extreme pain and make it to California. Of course, ever conscious of my "sit" time, I stand until the very last minute before departure.

An Asian man comes to the mike to announce boarding zones. At first he seems nondescript in his workman blue slacks and American West shirt, but then I notice the way he shifts so nimbly on the balls of his feet and immediately think he's a martial arts expert. His upper body is incredibly toned and his hips move loosely as he rotates with the small microphone in his hand. Later a short, soft, overweight white guy dressed in a shirt and tie makes a more important announcement about overbooked seats on the flight. The Asian fighter, clearly much lower on the employee totem pole, has a physical presence and fluidity Mr. Administrator could never match. As I hand Fighter Man my ticket, I'm even more impressed. He moves and looks like a serious athlete. There's not a spare ounce on his body.

Even more remarkable, I feel an immediate affinity for him, even though he barely registers me as I walk down the ramp. The simple fact he cares enough about his own physical being to stay in fantastic shape makes me want to know him. Of course that's not a whole lot different than connecting to someone simply because they have the same skin color as me. My blatant prejudice disturbs me. Many superbly fit people are incredibly egotistical and self-absorbed. Being in shape does not make them better than anyone else.

But I think I use fitness as a key social marker, just as I always scan the type of books people have in their homes. Both things say so much about the mind and body of the person I'm with. No books, well, that's a huge problem for me, especially if it's someone I want to date. A big gut, well, that's an even bigger problem. I know many people who struggle with their weight and exercise routines. I admit I speak understandingly to them but often feel bemused, an embarrassing fact about myself that I hope to confront at the Active Living Research Conference. As my man-in-the-street interviews in Washington, D.C. made clear, there are many reasons why people might not be active, reasons they cannot control. I definitely need a more open mind.

I land in San Diego without incident and without pain. My right hip rotates stiffly as I pull my luggage toward the car rental counter, but I feel nothing that a few Advil won't fix. For me, this is the most important segment of my road trip through America's sedentary culture. I have made it coast-to-coast in one day and I feel good. I grab my car keys already feeling like a Southern California beach blonde and head north along Route 5. I know I'm adding even more "sit" hours to my day, but I take my chances and stop at a state park for a hike and zip around to visit a cousin before finally settling at my final destination: the Marriott Hotel on Coronado Island. I have not experienced the ability to sit for long periods of time for years. I'm traveling across the country to find out more about getting people moving, yet I am ecstatic because I can sit for seven hours in one day.

On Friday morning I join a crowd of 300-plus people for breakfast and watch Dr. James Sallis, professor of psychology at San Diego State University and the program director for the Active Living Research Program, step to the podium in a lavender shirt and flashy tie. A trim, petite man with a huge smile and a cheerleader's pop, he welcomes us. Once again I am sitting, but I've had the night to rest and know there are all sorts of physical breaks worked into the program. This is, after all, a conference about movement.

I read a lot of Dr. Sallis' work before I arrived and like his blend of practical and academic solutions. He shows a sympathy I wish to acquire and believes the United States has created environments "that make it difficult to make healthful choices." The problems are so widespread and have built over so many decades that "programs promoting only personal responsibility will never be sufficient," he wrote in an editorial published in the *San Diego Tribune.* Change must come on many levels, he advocates, and the design and safety of built environments is an excellent place to start.

In some of his more academic work, he has chastised the various federal and nonprofit programs for being all over the map when it comes to suggested requirements: the USDA's Healthy People 2010 guidelines ask for thirty minutes of moderate activity a day, for example, while the National Association for Sports and Physical Education suggests at least sixty minutes. In one of his more technical papers written for the Georgia Health Policy Center, Dr. Sallis provides all sorts of nuts-and-bolts observations that have helped make him a media darling for reporters on the fitness beat. He writes:

- Physical education classes are not enough, and communities must also develop programs after school, especially outside.
- Family-centered activities don't work because parents are too crunched for time to make it.
- Crime rates have declined in the past fifteen years, but fear of crime has risen dramatically. It's such a problem that he believes that any new programs for kids in particular must include supervision as part of the package.
- Teenage girls and low-income minority youth are especially inactive and need special attention.
- Neighborhood design is one of the most important factors, next to safety, in encouraging physical activity in a local population.

Dr. Sallis has studied the problem of getting Americans moving again as long as any professional in the United States today, but at the conference he plays the emcee and soon hands the podium over to Terry Bazzare from the

Robert Wood Johnson Foundation, the nonprofit health research organization that funds most of the Active Living Research programs.

"Americans are on the move without moving," Dr. Bazzare says. The crowd of mostly middle-aged white people nods. A *Fortune* magazine cover flashes up on the PowerPoint screen on the stage: "Is FAT the Next Tobacco?" He follows this with a family tree of the Active Living Research programs, which includes Active Living by Design (the built environment), Active for Life (focuses on people fifty and older), Healthy Eating Research (obesity), and other departments. The tobacco connection is natural because the Robert Wood Johnson Foundation was very active in shaping the anti-smoking campaigns and wants to use many of the same formulas to address American's feeble activity levels and the country's battle with obesity.

The audience definitely seems jazzed by the time the first presenter comes to the mike, but things quickly quiet down as the various researchers present paper after paper on obvious things that it's hard to imagine scientists spending time and money to explore (hey, kids will play outside more if the parks are safe and close by) or on topics so narrow, like stair use in buildings, that it's clear the group is just talking among themselves and not doing a very effective job of reaching into the world where people apply ideas in real situations. At one point Dr. Sallis asked if there were any wellness program directors in the room and only a handful of people stood up. Most of the attendees are academics, architects, and urban planners.

Keith Laughlin of Rails and Trails had warned me that the ALR Conference might be a lot like the APHA meeting: lots of talk but few concrete plans for action. I decided to soldier on because as one presenter, Matt Coogan, told me at lunch, "You basically have most of the people in America who really want to find some answers all here in one place."

Coogan himself, who works for the New England Transportation Institute, raised some very interesting points in his presentation, which had the unwieldy title, "The Role of Neighborhood Form and Personal Values in the Determination of Walk and Transit Mode." In his research he found that if people really want to live in a walkable community and then do move to a walkable community, they *double* their activity level. Even people who rarely walk and care little about such things often increased their activity levels if they move to a walker-friendly place. Changes in the built environment can have a huge impact on even the most intractable, immobile American. If a family wants to walk, lives in a walkable community, *and* cuts back on the number of cars it owns, well, they become a regular tribe of trekkers.

At lunch, Coogan, a broad-faced, hefty man in his fifties, confided in me about his own personal struggle with weight. He was doing fine until they moved to a community where they had to drive everywhere to go to work, to get groceries, even to exercise. He put on thirty pounds. "You'd think walking up and down five flights of stairs to do the laundry would be enough," he laughs, referring to the layout of his new home.

I share with him that I had to cut three hours of intense full-court basketball games out of my week after my back surgery, but I replaced it with five days of moderate exercise, about an hour each day, and I managed to sustain my weight, though time remained a major problem. I feared he might think I was arrogant or self-congratulatory, but I was truly surprised that my approach had worked and told him so.

"Yeah, that will do it," he says, without a trace of ill feeling. "The [Robert Wood] Johnson Foundation is too focused on organized recreation. The real answer is in trying to get activity into the flow of the day."

The other talk I attended had a more catchy title and promised to get at the issue of will power that I found so difficult to pin down: "Do Americans Want Walkable Communities?" Dr. Susan Hardy from the University of California at Davis gave the presentation. An imposing, middle-aged white woman, she surveyed more than 5,000 people about several issues, including whether they wanted walkable communities. About 50 percent of the respondents said "yes." I felt that was like asking an obese person if they'd like to lose weight. Of course.

But try to measure what they are willing to do and to give up to achieve that goal and then the problems start. Would a family be willing to park its car half a mile away from their house so that the streets around their immediate neighborhood remained open for free play and pedestrians? And what about the 50 percent of people who couldn't even answer "yes" when asked if they wanted to be able to walk around more easily in their own neighborhood? Why was free and natural movement of so little importance in their life? How do we muster the political will for serious changes in the built environment when half of Americans claim they simply don't care?

I asked Dr. Hardy about measuring such things, and she insisted such issues were too abstract. She did say that her team of researchers found that if neighborhoods got too crowded that it could upset people. So access to stores, a library, or even a theater was good, but jamming too many people into a given walkable space is bad. Of course that's precisely what most "Smart Growth" advocates want to do, especially around urban metro stops.

At lunch I did meet up with Dr. Weimo Zhu, a Professor of Kinesiology at the University of Illinois at Urbana, who's hard at work on finding better ways to collect data, even on such abstract issues as political will. He's hoping to use things like cell phones that allow people to just dial in responses on a day-to-day basis instead of self-reporting questionnaires that are notoriously unreliable. Some of the presenters sent out thousands of forms for people to fill out but only got a return rate of less than 20 percent.

By the end of lunch, it's clear that the most popular "presenter" was Toni Yancey, a six-foot, African American woman, one-time college basketball player, and former model, who led the crowd through a "Liftoff L.A. Style." Her huge smile just radiated warmth, and she had everyone out of their seats in a matter of seconds. We all jogged in place and did a series of simple aerobic exercises with our arms.

"Palms to ceiling and now push," she says, raising her long limbs up and down to the music pumping in the background. Someone in the back knocks over a few glasses with his enthusiastic pushing and Yancey pokes fun at him.

"Really getting into it back there, huh?"

Everyone laughs and the entire chemistry of the room has gone from academic and cerebral to lighthearted and social in a matter of a minute. Dr. Sallis himself is up front whole-heartedly pumping his body in all directions. As I pushed and stepped, I felt the tension release in my hip, which was grateful for this socially acceptable chance to get up and just move. As the music faded and Yancey brought us all back down into our seats, she told the audience that this simple ten-minute workout actually lowered the blood pressure of employees who did it at the office. Small changes; good results.

So what if a community could start with a blank slate and tap into many of the excellent ideas circulating at the ALR conference? Is it possible to build a modern city or suburb that allows businesses to thrive even as people embrace a more physical daily life no longer centered on the car?

Well, Hurricane Katrina gave America its blank slate: New Orleans. On August 29, 2005, the Category 5 storm flooded two-thirds of the city when levees in certain key canals broke. Eleven hundred people died. Prior to the storm, 450,000 people lived there. Nearly all of them had to evacuate. Today thousands of homes sit abandoned. Large swaths of the city may never be resettled. New Orleans will probably never again have half-a-million residents.

A tall, thin man steps to the podium as the keynote speaker to tell us about what he's doing in New Orleans on a public-health level. I look down at my conference agenda and see, to my surprise, that it's none other than Rachel Wight's Dr. Tom Farley, public health professor at Tulane University in New Orleans and the co-author of *Prescription for a Healthy Nation*. The massive destruction opened up avenues for constructive change, he says, in a state that ranks forty-ninth in the nation for adult and infant mortality. The residents have average health insurance costs and average access to good healthcare, which means the real culprit is lifestyle related: alcohol, tobacco, diet, dismal physical-activity levels.

Using PowerPoint, Dr. Farley flashes a picture of a local convenience store on a street corner in New Orleans pre Katrina. A mix of handwritten signs and beer advertisements fill the windows. "Hotdogs, soda, cigarettes."

"You see a lot of this in New Orleans," Dr. Farley says, his slight frame leaning against the podium. "But not this."

A slide of a grocery produce section filled with fresh vegetables pops up.

"A 1970s' marketing survey found that if you gave fruits and vegetables twice the space in a grocery store, it would generate a 40 percent increase in sales. You don't even need an educational program, just increased space."

A picture of rows and rows of soda on supermarket shelves replaces the veggie photo.

"Accessibility is just a huge problem."

For the next few minutes, the audience sees images of a Burger King and McDonald's within walking distance of a New Orleans high school, more convenience stores plugging junk food and liquor, pizza joints, and, the crowd favorite, a drive-through Daiquiri Shop.

"I think this is unique to New Orleans," Dr. Farley quips. "You don't even need to get out of your car to get an alcoholic drink." Everyone laughs.

Nearly every major player involved in public health and city planning in the nation converged on New Orleans with ideas on what to do post-Katrina. The Urban Land Institute, a nonprofit that specializes in "creating better places," suggested New Orleans shrink the footprint of the city and cut off the most vulnerable areas along the levees. The Institute wanted many old neighborhoods converted to parkland, but, of course, most of the former residents were poor and African American, so many called foul and claimed discrimination.

People like Dr. Farley advocated for rebuilding communities that required residents to walk rather than drive. There was talk of penalizing stores for selling unhealthy food and giving tax breaks to grocers who sold more fruits and vegetables. Others laid out a beautiful blueprint for a light transit system that would discourage people from driving.

The audience at the ALR Conference, desperately looking for success stories, let the words wash over them like Southern California sunlight: Smartshrinking! Tax breaks for healthy foods! Light transit!

Then Dr. Farley recounted his experience sitting in on a local neighborhood association meeting with the director of public works for New Orleans. They had come to discuss the light rail. The director made it clear that prior to Hurricane Katrina he had 250 staffers. Since the storm he had laid off 200 of them. He promised citizens in the room that the city would get stop signs up at all of the intersections that had broken traffic lights. He wasn't sure if he had the resources to deal with the horrible pothole problem.

They never got around to discussing the light rail. Two days later the director resigned.

On September 15, 2005, President George Bush pledged $200 billion toward the rebuilding of New Orleans, but in the next few months the amount dropped somewhere closer to the range of $6 billion. Louisiana Governor Kathleen Blanco decided to spend the bulk of the money to buy out homes of displaced residents, which didn't leave a whole lot left for things like light transit.

"The city is in financial collapse," Dr. Farley says. "Three thousand city officials have been laid off, so essentially there's no functioning government." And the governor, mayor, urban planning board, local neighborhood associations, local city council, and various federal agencies are all having turf battles. There's no central clearinghouse for ideas and no clear person or commission with the power to make final decisions.

At least most of the people involved in the conversation remain interested in keeping New Orleans a walkable city, says Dr. Farley, but "things like access to healthy food just fly over planners' heads. It's too abstract and refined an idea for them."

The room is very, very, very quiet. The California Sunshine has left the building.

Dr. Sallis, ever the upbeat emcee, skips onto the podium and says, "We'd all help in someway if we could." But, of course, we can't.

"There's no substitute for competent, efficient government, no matter how many brilliant ideas there might be in the private sector," Dr. Farley concludes. "You'll always bump up against the government."

Later, after this conference, he and some of his colleagues at Tulane actually teamed up with the CDC and, in 2007, created the Partnership for an Active Community Environment (PACE), which is using the hard-hit and poverty stricken upper Ninth Ward of New Orleans as a lab for new ideas. How much will even the most disadvantaged Americans change their dietary habits if the local markets offer a lot more fresh produce at reasonable prices? How much more active will the locals be if their public spaces are well-lighted, cleaned up, and close by? How much can group counseling work to get at the root of certain behaviors, such as poor eating habits or a sedentary lifestyle? What happens if we make the physical changes in their environment *and* provide emotional counseling at the same time? PACE is trying out all of these ideas and looking at the answers over a five-year period ending in 2012.

But Dr. Farley does not mention any of this in his keynote address because PACE is just in its infancy, so I leave the room once again feeling that a lot of ideas are getting swirled around like the beer foam in the glass I'm drinking out of at a bar at the end of the evening. Here I am on a vital step in my journey to track the broken American body. I had finally fixed my own body to the point where I could make the trip, and, still, most of what I hear from the experts is just talk.

A slight woman with brown-gray hair to her shoulders, eyeglasses, and a distinctly practical (rather than beachy) East Coast look walks by my table. We give each other a second look, and I realize that she must be Sharon Roerty, executive director for the National Center for Bicycling & Walking, whom I've been trying to find all weekend. I'm not sure why I know it's Sharon out of the hundreds of people at the conference, but the fact I know she hails from New Jersey and she's about my age certainly helped. I invite her to join me.

I feel an instant rapport with this no-nonsense, fit, middle-aged woman who speaks freely and candidly about anything I bring up. She cycled all around the island today, she tells me, as we bite into our sandwiches. The program she directs sends staffers on location to cities and suburbs all across the country. They work with existing personnel and existing infrastructure to find ways to increase bicycling and walking in various communities. Of course the center will always push for new trails when they can, but the resources for such things aren't always there, so the staffers work hard to adapt to whatever reality presents itself.

She tells me a terrific story about Louisville, Kentucky, where they worked with a Democratic district to create a popular biking program. A Republican candidate from a neighboring district, eager to keep up with a party rival, wanted his constituents to have the same program. Then long-time Mayor Dave Abramson, decided to get involved as well and launched a program, "Healthy Hometown Hike and Bike," and hired a bicycle-pedestrian coordinator. He used his considerable political weight to recruit local businesses to get involved financially and physically in the campaign. In May 2005, Louisville had its first official "Healthy Hometown Hike and Bike" event. A thousand people participated in the fourteen-mile bike ride along the river. In February 2006, *Men's Health* magazine ranked Louisville ninth on its list of "Fit Cities in the United States," in large part because of Abramson's aggressive political agenda on biking and fitness. In general, Louisville residents are actually heavier and less active than the national average, but there's been measurable improvements in the activity levels of the locals since Abramson began pushing the bike trails and related programs.

"Envy is a great tool," Sharon says with a laugh that somehow has a New Jersey accent.

I confess to her how discouraged I feel sometimes about bringing about substantive, system-wide changes. To my relief, she puts me in my place.

"Hey, there's always hope. I can go to a place where the landscape is decimated and there's no political interest, but there's one person on the city staff that cares about bike trails, and, well, you'd be amazed what one enthused person can do. At least all of that stuff [about access to healthy food and walkability] was included in the planning discussions [in New Orleans]. That's just incredible."

Her optimism begins to take hold inside of me as well.

"The Bush administration is not interested in any of this, but all of these issues continue to be discussed on a national level anyway. They can't ignore the sheer volume of concern. There's a real groundswell."

I tell her about sitting next to a man on the airplane on the way to San Diego who was reading *Making the Nation Safe: The Role of Science and Technology in Countering Terrorism*, published by the National Research Council. I get so frustrated by all of the money and time spent on national security when one of the greatest threats to the collective citizenry is America's lifestyle habits.

"Yeah," she says, "and how did the people who survived the Twin Towers get out? They walked out. In New Orleans there were tons of stories of people walking and biking out, even though officials actually tried to close roads to pedestrian traffic."

I admit, I had never thought of it in that light, but Americans' inability to walk five miles at a decent pace could wind up being a major national security issue. We can't always expect to be able to flee by car, airplane, train, or bus. In the end, if something really awful happens, like the attack on the Twin Towers, it's the people who can rely on their own physical selves who will survive and get where they need to go.

If you can't walk five miles, you're a national security risk to your country. Who would ever have the guts to say something so radical?

By the time I leave the bar, Sharon Roerty has got me thinking in a whole new way. There's hope in places I never expected and tools I never thought to tap into (security and envy!). I decide I want to know more about what landscapes and street dynamics work best and will trek through one of the most walkable cities in the United States, New York City, with my new guide, Sharon Roerty. Leave it to a Jersey girl to have some clever, street-wise answers.

10

The Social Costs

Trekking New York City for Answers

When I was in grammar school in the late 1960s, 50 percent of kids biked to school; today less than 1 percent do. Somewhere in that thirty-five-year span, Americans stopped feeling comfortable moving through public spaces. They came to prefer their cars, homes, offices, indoor exercise rooms, and organized daycare centers. Each weekday morning fewer than one in eight school-age children set off for class on foot, even though the majority live within a mile of their public school.

Of course walking eight to ten blocks at a moderate pace doesn't burn off many calories so I'm not sure how much this cultural change has directly contributed to the rise in obesity, but it does reflect a general drift toward a more sedentary attitude and has had profound *social* consequences.

By the time I was ten, I confidently navigated my neighborhood alone, enjoyed hours of free play each day near a local stream, and regularly shopped in stores without adult supervision. My teenage daughter does walk around a local mall with her friends on occasion, but has yet to experience anything remotely like the moments I once had around Trout Brook in Connecticut. This delayed exposure to unfettered movement in public areas has definitely hurt her social development. She's a better student than I ever was, but lacks the confident independence I had acquired by fifth grade.

I blame the way American society constantly gets in the way of children's physical freedom. The lack of pedestrian traffic in most areas, especially suburbs, makes the streets seem like hollow tubes. The emptiness encourages more emptiness and fear.

Families will agree to carpool but not bike-pool because the local roads lack safe bicycle lanes. On several key stretches of the three-mile journey between my house and my daughter's former middle school, there are no sidewalks. I'm so passionate about getting Americans moving again that I spent three years writing this book, but I *still* had to drive my child to middle school. The local landscape and culture make it very difficult to choose any other option. When we slash physical movement out of our daily commutes, we interact less with the general community. We see the people we choose to see and who look the most like us. When my daughter rides in my car to school, she sees the back of my head and the front lawns of her well-to-do neighbors.

I spent a week observing children leaving local elementary and middle schools in Alexandria and Arlington, Virginia. I knew Arlington, in particular, had won an urban planning award after spending millions of dollars on improvements that made the areas between neighborhoods and public schools more pedestrian friendly. I saw the speed bumps, new sidewalks, slower speed limits, and better signage. But I'm afraid that even in Arlington the overall average is about two walkers for every ten kids. The Arlington County website claims that at some of the elementary schools 100 percent of the kids walk home, but what they really mean is that 100 percent of the kids COULD walk, since they live a mile or less from the school. Measuring the number of kids who ACTUALLY walk is an altogether different story.

To really understand the social consequences of our physically confining lives, I needed a place where more people move around by walking through their local landscape. Many travel magazines and organizations, like the American Podiatric Medical Association, publish lists of "The Top Ten Most Walkable Cities." Portland, Oregon, and Seattle, Washington, generally rank in the top two, but I knew I needed something bigger, grittier, and more spontaneous. I knew I needed New York City. And who better to lead the way than a native of the New Jersey-New York border and a national expert on getting people back into public spaces, Sharon Roerty.

Despite her slight build and soft brown hair, I see her immediately when I exit the Newark train station after a four-hour ride from Washington, D.C. She's leaning against her black Volvo, which has two bicycles on the roof.

"Ready to ride?" she asks, with a smile and a wave.

I had forgotten that she wanted to do a short bicycle tour of the waterfront in New Jersey before we set off for Manhattan the next morning, but I'm happy for the chance to loosen my back and right hip.

We drive through a stressed neighborhood in Newark strewn with broken things and clumps of edgy men on corners. I feel conspicuous in our station wagon with bikes, but Sharon looks completely unfazed. As executive director of the National Center for Bicycling & Walking, she regularly travels to precisely these kinds of down-and-out places to talk about how to get healthier and more vibrant traffic on the sidewalks. More eyes, less crime; less crime, more business; more business, less trash and busted buildings. It's a pretty simple equation in her eyes.

We pull into Jersey State Park. A firm breeze stirs up waves on the Hudson River and catches me in the face. The fine spring Sunday afternoon has brought out all sorts of boat traffic on the river and human traffic on the boardwalk, which is about ten feet wide, flat, and right along the water's edge. I settle into the bicycle Sharon has brought for me and follow her at a slow roll as we move through the stream of people: Africans, Indians, Latin Americans, Asians. The backside of the Statue of Liberty comes into view, and we laugh about the fact that people in Jersey get to see the statue's ass.

Ellis Island comes up on our right.

While we pass several signs that warn, "Hazardous Waste Keep Out," in general the state has transformed this former marsh and rundown industrial park into an impressive recreational area. There's a large playground, lots of green fields for free play, and a fantastic view of the river. I love the loose mood of the place (no organized sports games going on here) and of my guide, who, despite her work for a national bicycling organization, is not a fanatic who needs to ride 100 miles a day. Sharon's not motivated by cool equipment, competitive races, or a desire for six-pack abs.

"It's all about getting movement into the flow of everyday life," she tells me.

As we continue our Jersey Park tour, she talks about cycling this area and the city as a kid.

"I had friends who were bus-route friends and others that were biking friends or walking-distance friends. My bus-route friends would stick their hands out the window and wave at me so I'd know what bus to take." Sharon laughs. Her face still has a girlish flair to it, especially her smile. I laugh with her and think about how she built a layered social life by varying the way she moved through the cityscape, something kids today would have trouble understanding.

We pull onto another boardwalk and ride past a rusted steel girder, now part of a 9/11 memorial, which came from the fallen World Trade Center Towers that once stood directly across the Hudson River. Trees line that section of Manhattan's waterfront now. We stop.

"I watched all of the stages of [construction] of the Trade Center Towers," she says. "My dad brought us to see the huge hole they dug [for the foundation], and later we went back several times so we could watch it being built. My dad loved all forms of moving around—by boat, tunnel, train, on foot. He tried all varieties. Maybe that was a factor in my getting interested in transportation. 'Today let's go by tunnel,' he'd say. Next time it might be the rail. He showed us all the different ways you could move around."

He died ten years ago, but she mentions him often during our tour.

Sharon, who normally projects enormous amounts of positive social energy, becomes subdued as we look at where the World Trade Center Towers once stood. But just as quickly she shrugs off the feeling, swings her bicycle back into action, and continues an upbeat monologue about Jersey City, her relatives who came through Ellis Island (and made it no further than across the river), and her cravings for chocolate milk when she was pregnant.

I see now the spirit that sustains her when she travels to cities like Baltimore and St. Louis and faces tremendous skepticism when she talks about all the ways even the most blighted neighborhoods can improve foot traffic on sidewalks and in public parks. She preaches all over the country about the importance of adding movement into the flow of the average American life, which, in turn, will dramatically enhance the social connections of people in communities; sometimes only a handful of locals show up to listen. But in her mind, all she needs is the ear of one engaged person and she's made an inroad into a new place.

We close our bicycle ride at the parking lot and drive to Sharon's house in Maplewood, New Jersey, where her two teenage kids and husband await us for dinner. Tomorrow we head to Manhattan, this time on foot.

The next morning, we strap on our pedometers, which measure the number of footsteps a person takes in a day, and head out for the train. As we stride through the established residential neighborhood, lined with old trees and houses with porches, we follow the same path to the station that her son and daughter walk each day to school. She takes great pride in the fact that they travel on foot most days.

Maplewood itself is a thriving small town complete with several blocks of locally owned businesses (no chain stores here), a large public park, and a classic turn-of-the-century train depot. More than forty people have parked their bicycles outside, a good showing in a town of 22,000 (there's fewer than a dozen bikes most days at my metro station in Alexandria, a town of 140,000).

Inside the train station, we join a racially diverse but economically homogenous line of commuters waiting to buy tickets. People must have good jobs to live this close to New York in such a quaint and walkable town. I think back to the section of Newark we drove through. Clearly living near safe public spaces is increasingly becoming a privilege for the affluent and few, not a communal right.

Once on the train, Sharon points out the center of South Orange as we roll past.

"They used to have four lanes of traffic, and people used their cars just to cross the street," she says. But Sharon and other urban planners worked with the local government and had them widen the sidewalks, narrow the street to two lanes, and impose much lower speed limits. Pedestrian traffic increased dramatically.

We chat about the ultimate guru of walkable communities, Jane Jacobs, who died in 2006 at age eighty-nine. Jacobs' hugely influential book, *The*

Death and Life of Great American Cities, which came out in 1961, aggressively challenged the tendency among urban planners of the 1950s and 1960s to level old sections of cities to make way for glossy high rises and open, dramatic spaces, like the Lincoln Center. She led an exhausting but successful fight against New York kingpin builder, Robert Moses, who wanted to put an expressway through the residential neighborhood now commonly known as SoHo. Jacobs, who lived on Hudson Street in Greenwich Village at the time, got so emotional at one point that she and several others stormed the podium at a City Planning Commission meeting. A few years later she got herself arrested for "criminal mischief" because she disrupted another public meeting about the construction of the highway, which, thanks in part to such antics, never got built.

In *The Death and Life of Great American Cities*, Jacobs talks about the importance of eyes on the street, on the casual but regular contact of strangers in public spaces, on living in neighborhoods that sustain a human scale. In many ways, her book celebrates the role casual *physical* activity—walking, biking, lounging at the local café—plays in people's *social* lives.

In the obituaries I read about her, I learned that Jacobs loved to "talk" out loud to Thomas Jefferson and Benjamin Franklin everyday and used her conversations with the two men to help her wrestle ideas to the page. (Personally, I'd favor Jefferson.) She never finished college and worked variously as a secretary, candy factory worker, and freelance writer. She used her pen to break out of her confining life and to carry her ideas to some satisfying conclusions, a quest I can relate to as I sit next to Sharon and discuss city and suburban landscapes in America.

In recent decades, urban planners have carried many of Jacobs' ideas to the extreme under the rubric "New Urbanism," which itself morphed into something called "Smart Growth" (an oxymoron in my dictionary). In an effort to stop sprawl, Smart Growth advocates pushed for dense development zones in places like Portland, Oregon, and Arlington, Virginia (outside of Washington, D.C.). The idea was to cram as many people as possible around subways and bus routes instead of in sprawling suburban communities that rely too heavily on the car. On many levels it makes sense, but in terms of crafting more inviting public spaces it does not. All around me in Northern Virginia I see huge stands of high-rise apartments (with the same, flat-faced boring brick design) dominating city streets that may have sidewalks, but so little genuine human culture and life that it's no fun to walk there.

I feel the same way about contrived small towns like Reston, Virginia, where developers plopped a town green, sidewalks, and small shops into a box-shaped plan surrounded by parking lots. They think they created an old-fashioned neighborhood, but whenever I go there, I feel as though I'm walking through a movie set.

I don't mention any of this to Sharon. It's just white noise in my mind as we sit in silence. But it does bring home to me how complicated it can be to undo the damage caused by sprawl and to craft landscapes that people will want to return to in a physical sense.

Our train passes through the Meadowlands and Sharon begins talking about something called SAFETYLU. She spells it out for me, and it's actually SAFETEA-LU, an abbreviation for a new federal government program that has allocated $612 million for Safe Routes to Schools (SRS) programs across the country.

"It's really about youth mobility," she says.

What incredible news. The federal government has decided to throw tax dollars at something as abstract as getting kids to physically move through their communities again. Wow. I want to hug Sharon and bang on the seat in front of me, but I just nod my head. Sharon herself will be involved with how New Jersey spends its share of the SRS money, which will include building trails, bicycle lanes on main roads, more sidewalks, and traffic "calming" measures. In the sample pilot program in Marin County, California, the percentage of kids walking to school shot up 64 percent in just two years.

Of course walking a mile isn't going to make a ten-year-old physically fit, but it could make her more confident about navigating things on her own, get her parent's car off the road in the morning, and get her blood moving before school starts, which will help her concentrate.

Sharon and I debark at Penn Station and catch a subway to the first neighborhood on my list: the Lower East Side, which was the most densely populated area in the western world at the turn of the century. Largely known as a center for Eastern European Jews, the neighborhood actually had waves of different groups, starting in the early nineteenth century with Germans, then

Irish, and, later, Italians. Today there's a sizable Dominican population and, of course, still many Jews.

A tribal mentality governed the place; whole villages from places like Belarus relocated to a specific street or even a specific group of houses. With so little personal space within the tenements, everyone had to circulate in public.

We emerge near Delancy Street. Most of the five-story, narrow homes have been sandblasted clean. Instead of strong smells and loud chatter from street vendors, we see flower pots on fire escapes and a Starbucks.

"There goes the neighborhood," Sharon says with a light smile as she points out the coffee shop. Of course she's not entirely serious because the tight streets, old homes, and general lay of the neighborhood still provide a glove-like intimacy. I can just see neighbors shouting across to each other from the upper-story windows. After all, Starbucks—the only chainstore I see—is a coffee shop where people gather.

High rents have transformed this area. Jews still dominate the cultural scene, but we need to head to Chinatown to fully feel the "teeming masses" of immigrants moving through New York City streets.

As we travel west, the pedestrian traffic thickens and the smells become more pungent, like a musky greenhouse. Starting in the 1980s, hundreds of thousands of Chinese—again, whole villages—immigrated to the U.S, which helps account for why Chinatown now threatens to swallow everything around it, including Little Italy and portions of the Lower East Side. I hear clips of conversation, probably in Cantonese or Mandarin (perhaps even Fujianese).

Something other than crowded living spaces pushes these people into the streets. They brought with them certain habits with regard to public areas, such as a common well or village square, which made them comfortable mingling outside, a quality most Americans have lost. (In fact, even the word "mingling" seems so dated.) Dozens of slight Asian men work steadily to move huge wooden plats loaded with bags of onions or potatoes. Mothers sit by their baby carriages in the local park. Old men lean on full burlap sacks watching the street scene. I see signs for dozens of noodle shops: Hung Kai Noodle, Wing Kei Noodle. Many people here never leave this place or learn to speak English or ever own a car. This is most certainly not Reston, Virginia. There's no parking lot in sight.

Sustaining a brisk walking pace, Sharon and I pass over into Little Italy. After Chinatown, it feels cleaner but more touristy and less authentic. We press on, a bit tired from the street noise, the endless stream of people that somehow pass us but rarely bump, and settle down for a cup of coffee on a bench in SoHo, close by Jane Jacobs' old neighborhood.

So this is what she saved: blocks and blocks of splendid five-story apartment houses with cast-iron fire escapes out front and a necklace-like strand of local restaurants and funky stores interspersed throughout. Some critics claim that the place has become a gentrified tourist and yuppie haven and no longer has the neighborhood soul that Jacobs' so celebrated, but the scale for the pedestrian is ideal. I'm happy to pause here. The slant of sunlight from above enhances the intimacy of the space. I see lots of motorized scooters and tube-tire bicycles locked up on various side streets. I don't see any chainstores, and there's plenty of foot traffic; not as dense as Chinatown, but steady and vibrant.

Sharon sips coffee and tells me that she plans to retire to Manhattan.

"I want to grow old where I can walk even if I don't know anyone. When I get out I want to feel part of something; to be in the flow of people." Her own mother lives in subdivision isolation somewhere in Texas, which stresses Sharon to no end.

"I gotta get her out of there."

We move on through the Greenwich Village area, past landmark bars, like the Red Lion and the Bottom Line, where artists like Bruce Springsteen and Bob Dylan first made their names. This feels more like fraternity row, which makes sense since New York University sits just across the way. We settle down again at Washington Square Park, where Sharon begins to open up about her work and her feelings about movement and community life in America.

"We need to remind people what they like. They forget. They like sharing open spaces and seeing neighbors." She brings up her mother again, who spent most of her adult life in urban places like Jersey City and New York, but now lives down in Bush country in Texas. "People need something besides the weather to talk about. It's so sterile. [We] need a little mischief around to feel alive."

We both look at the "mischief" going on around us in this typical New York City park, complete with curved sidewalks that encourage people to sit on the benches rather than walk a straight line through the space. Kids play behind a fenced-in playground. Lots of students study while sitting on the grass and listening to their iPods. An old woman observes people.

Sharon really opens up now and begins talking with feeling about her work. Staffers from the National Center for Bicycling & Walking only go into communities where they are invited. "We don't get grants to spread the word of God," as Sharon explains it with a laugh. "We go where they want us."

They go in pairs to places like Baltimore. She describes the two experiences she had there, one in the city and the other in the suburbs in Baltimore County.

"I just loved the series we did in Baltimore City. I could see that the people were struggling. They talked about putting flowers on the streets and the kids would just ruin them. So I said, well, just move the flowers to the windowsills on the second floor. Leave the lights on. Add things that work to make your sidewalks a more inviting place. I understand their fears and know how to work with what they do have.

"But Baltimore County was dreadful to me. They thought they had pedestrian friendly places. They had a big brick plaza that had 'No Loitering' and 'No Skateboarding' signs all over it. It reminded me of the plastic covers on the furniture that some of the moms used when we were kids. Heavy plastic slip covers. I mean they had bumpy pavement, which is no good for bikes or wheelchairs, fountains that didn't allow swimming. I sat in that room and only a few people from the community even bothered to come."

So the struggling low-income crowd in the city had the personal commitment, but few resources and legitimate concerns about safety. The Baltimore County crowd had the cash and quiet, but no public will. But Sharon keeps on traveling to make her point and often has the most success in the most desperate areas because "it's not about the money, it's about the commitment. Things are not that expensive. Streets have a ten-year life cycle so just put the changes into the master plan. If you're going to repave anyway, then add bike lanes and wider sidewalks and make the local government, not just the engineers, help put the plan in place."

We're scheduled to meet my mother and stepfather, who are in their eighties, for lunch at a restaurant off 42nd Street, so we set out again; our pedometers have registered 17,000-plus steps so far. Of course Times Square and the theater district are not neighborhoods as much as happening spaces. Everything is huge: the flashing billboards, the street traffic, the cost of T-shirts. We thread through a volume of walkers unlike anything I ever experience back home in Washington, D.C., which is a good-sized city in its own right, but feels like a plain white dinner plate next to New York's street fare.

My mother, a petite woman with green eyes and remarkably lush white hair, continues to thrive in her eighties in part because she's such an avid walker. She and my stepfather travel all over the world, and wherever she goes she engages in the local landscape by walking through it. She visits open markets, talks to strangers, strolls beaches, and visits offbeat shops. For many years, when they traveled to American Bar Association meetings across the country, she had a group of women from the ABA crowd who walked with her, but many became ill, had falls, or lost a spouse so stopped coming to events. Most of the time she walks alone now. I think of Sharon and how she wants to retire in Manhattan and think of how successfully my mother has sustained a thriving social life, even when walking alone, because each time she strikes out she inserts herself into the larger community—exactly what Sharon envisions for herself when she grows old.

After lunch we head out for the final leg of our Manhattan tour, Central Park, which a journalist once described as "the single greatest work of art in the city of New York." It took twenty years and thousands of men to shape the 843-acre canvas into the remarkable public space visitors see today. Back in the 1850s, when city officials and residents began to first seriously talk about setting aside land for a public park, no other city in America had anything like what Frederick Law Olmsted, the park's superintendent, and his partner, English-born architect Calvert Vaux, presented in their proposed design, often referred to as the Greensward Plan. They didn't want an amusement park. They wanted an uplifting open space where city residents could go for quiet and stress-reducing open vistas and wooded glens. They wanted pedestrian traffic, not carriages, to dominate, and even designed dozens of small bridges that forced vehicle traffic overhead while walkers could stroll underneath.

Many of the city's laborers and immigrants favored an amusement park and playing fields for competitive games and felt the European flair of the

Greensward Plan catered to the wealthy and would discourage the average city resident from using the public space. The two sides argued in the newspapers and in the courts but, backed by many of the wealthy homeowners that faced the potential park (and would see their house values skyrocket), Olmsted and Vaux's plan won.

One of their counterarguments: the huge immigrant class would finally have somewhere else to go after work besides the bars. And they did come. By the 1860s more than three million people were visiting the park on foot every year and another four million by horse carriage.

The success of Central Park inspired other cities in the United States to set aside sizable portions of their landscapes for public parks on a grand scale, including Hartford, Connecticut; Baltimore, Maryland; Brooklyn, New York; and others. The New Yorkers pulled it off during a severe economic depression in the mid-nineteenth century, which just further underscores Sharon's point that commitment, not money, really lies at the heart of the matter. Indeed one of the biggest upgrades in the history of Central Park took place during the Great Depression in the 1930s. The more stressful city life became, the more the city government and citizens safeguarded their illustrious park.

Sharon and I travel down 7th Avenue past the Carousel ($1.50 a ride) and watch a horse-drawn carriage cross over the bridge on Transverse Avenue. It's late afternoon on a Monday and the park is absolutely packed. We're headed to what Sharon likes to call the "urban beach," which is actually Sheep's Meadow.

The swirly sidewalks encourage a people-watching pace. Sharon snaps lots of pictures. A couple comes over and asks her to please remove the photographs of them from her camera because it violates their religion. Sharon doesn't miss a beat and shows them the digital file on the camera and deletes it. They smile; she shakes her head and they part. I can't help but think that all of her movement through public spaces in this area honed the social skills that made that scene no scene for her. She doesn't even mention it as we continue our walk, whereas most suburban kids I know would have felt really threatened.

We walk up a hill to a fence and a collection of basalt rocks that overlook Sheep's Meadow, a great green expanse crowded with mothers and their babies, workers taking a break, and college kids throwing Frisbees and footballs.

Actually Olmsted felt that people shouldn't even walk on Sheep's Meadow, just contemplate it while the animals grazed. The people won and the sheep are gone, but it still remains a free space, not confined by backstops for baseball fields or lines for soccer fields. No one needs a special permit to use this area.

Sharon mentions Baltimore County again. "They just don't get it," she says.

But mostly we're quiet. At this point our pedometers read nearly 25,000 steps.

I could never live in Manhattan; too over-stimulating. Yet my visit called up feelings of longing and restlessness. At the time I made this trip to New York City, I lived on a cul-de-sac within a mile of a metro, a park, and a historic commercial district, but it was still a social dead-end. Nine kids under the age of thirteen lived in a fifteen-house area, but none of them played in the common spaces (street, sidewalk, or front lawns). In New York, I felt my place in the stream of humanity; in Alexandria, I felt an aloneness that only dissolved if I deliberately sought out "mischief."

I would never want Alexandria to be a mini-Manhattan, but Sharon has become an expert at working with what's already on hand in communities. She understands she's really drumming up an *emotional* commitment to rebuild communal spaces through movement by challenging Americans' sedentary lifestyles. My cul-de-sac could easily have been as busy as Sheep's Meadow, of course on a scale that makes sense for nine kids.

On the way home we decide we want to stop for a beer at a bar in Maplewood where the locals like to go after snowstorms to spontaneously share a draft. Over dinner she observes that we never once had to climb over a highway barrier, wall, or cross a huge highway.

"The thing about New York City, especially Manhattan, is that it all works. It's not some Disneyland, made-up community. It's a string of real neighborhoods."

I agree but say little. For now I need to just sit back and think about it all.

But days later, when I am home by my stand-up desk, I come to a very surprising conclusion. Prior to my New York trip, I spent months reading books like Jane Jacobs' *Death and Life of Great American Cities*, *Asphalt Nation:*

How the Automobile Took Over America and How We Can Take It Back by Jane Kay, *The Geography of Nowhere: The Rise and Decline of America's Man-made Landscape* by James Kunstler, and *Downtown* by Peter Hamill. I researched online about Safe Routes to Schools programs and publications put out by the National Center for Bicycling & Walking. I educated myself about the history of urban planning, the general trends and problems facing suburbs and cities today. I interviewed experts.

But in the end, the most worthwhile insight came in an e-mail Sharon sent me a few days after our New York tour. She shared something inside of her that no book author or urban-planning specialist can measure, but which we all need if we hope to turn the corner and break free from the most damaging aspects of our sedentary culture.

She wrote: "I do what I do because I am afraid to live in a world without community life. I'm afraid to leave my children in a world with no sidewalks. I want you to promise me that the chapter that includes me is about people and hope and a love of community life."

11

A Spiritual Solution?

What sort of community will we have if we keep going on the path that we're on? What will happen to our bodies, our social lives, our landscapes, our kids? Imagine living in a neighborhood where 50 percent of the children eventually develop Type 2 diabetes, where 40 percent of the adults never exercise, or where people suffer from cancer, stress, heart disease, and obesity at rates that make the national average look tame.

Many Hispanics and African Americans live in that "neighborhood," and it's not a hypothetical place for them. These numbers are the real averages for these groups in the United States. Allowing the trends to continue uninterrupted is a form of racism on par with denying citizens the vote, access to housing, or good schools. It's created a horrible sore in the underbelly of our collective health, a wound that we must heal if we hope to regain our national vigor.

Some studies show that certain people from a variety of racial and ethnic backgrounds may be genetically predisposed to "hold" weight. In cultures that often went through lean times, this advantage could have been the difference between survival and death. But even if such a link proves valid, it would only account for maybe 10 percent of the obesity and other health-related issues among Hispanics and African Americans, which means the other 90-plus percent has to do with education, environment, and resources.

People who live in neighborhoods they consider unsafe are *four times* as likely to be obese. They may have public parks within walking distance, but they aren't going there. They may have a local gym where they could play basketball, but they aren't going there. They stay in their apartments, in front of their TVs, and only go outside if they have to work.

And when they do venture out, they often must move through landscapes that offer few safe spaces for pedestrian traffic: six-to-eight lane highways with crossing lights that don't work, poor (or no) sidewalks, and bus stops at illogical places. Low-income Hispanics, in particular, have a habit of compounding the poor conditions with risky walking patterns.

I've read about it in studies, but I've also seen it firsthand by the dealership where I get my car repaired, which is located in a lower-income neighborhood. If I arrive in the morning, I see dozens of Hispanic adults crossing Route 1—a six-lane highway—at all angles and places to get to the bus stop in front of the dealership. They dodge one car, stand on the line of the next lane until a car brushes by going forty-five to fifty miles per hour, then move to the next line, as though the fading white paint is some sort of safe bubble.

When I come in the late afternoon, I see young mothers pushing their babies in strollers using the same dodge-from-line-to-line technique. Each time I visit the dealership, there's a notice posted at the bus stop pleading in both English and Spanish for pedestrians to use the official crosswalks. Often there's a news announcement as well about someone who was killed by a car while walking in the area.

But when I look left and right, I see that the nearest crossing light is almost a half-a-mile away in either direction. This combination of poor urban planning and cultural habits has meant that Hispanics get hit by cars while walking more than any other group in the United States.

This is *fear* and *lack* on a scale that most of us can't even imagine.

The hard fact is that many African Americans and Hispanics eat too much and move too little. They struggle with this deadly equation even more than their white and Asian counterparts. It's easy to claim that they need to take more personal responsibility for their health (we all do); that's certainly a valid assertion. But Americans also need to look at factors that enable unhealthy lifestyle habits. For example, social researchers have found that Hispanics who live in neighborhoods that have grocers that carry their native foods have far fewer weight problems, but how many urban planners or zoning boards know that?

In places like the pricey historic district in Alexandria, Virginia, where I lived for ten years, there are zoning laws and tax laws that protect and buffer locally run businesses so the national chain stores, with their deep pockets, won't swoop in and transform the quirky, historic shopping strip into another outdoor mall. The same approach could be used to safeguard ethnic grocery stores in low-income neighborhoods, which might be threatened by a Mc-Donald's or Wendy's.

At the Active Living Research Conference I attended in San Diego, the keynote speaker, Dr. Farley of Tulane University, talked about taking this very approach in low-income African American communities in New Orleans. He flashed slide after slide of grocers in poor neighborhoods that carried plenty of beer, chips, soda, and hot dogs, but almost no fresh produce. Now many of these places were family-run businesses, so being locally owned is hardly a cure-all. Instead Dr. Farley suggested an even more targeted incentive: tax breaks for offering healthier food choices on the shelves. And, as he pointed out, studies show that if a grocer doubles the amount of produce on her floor, the locals will double the amount of fruits and vegetables they purchase and eat.

While access plays a huge role in healthy diets, most low-income minorities cite safety and time as their two main concerns when it comes to exercise. Yet even among these overworked populations, the average person has twenty-eight to thirty hours of leisure a week. So why can't they find four or five hours a week to move their bodies? The answer lies in a place where studies rarely go, in the spirit and energy a person carries through their day. If you work two jobs to live in a crime-ridden area and must endure long commutes from bus-to-bus to get where you need to go, then any "spare" time you have is just an illusion. You arrive home so spent you long for passive leisure, like television.

Public schools make some effort to provide more for the children in these difficult neighborhoods; but even there, few programs actually listen to what their student population really wants or needs. In one study of African American and white middle school girls at a public urban school, researchers found that white students liked more organized activities, such as ballet, soccer, and softball, and spent more of their time outside of school doing homework. The African American girls liked dancing, basketball, TV, and church.

Schools tend to offer more activities that white children prefer. The end result, African American girls have much lower self-esteem when it comes to physical activity than their white counterparts. If gym class only offers softball and you like to dance, well . . .

I remember where I grew up in Connecticut in the 1970s all of the girls' gym classes centered on gymnastics. I could barely touch my toes, even at age ten, and kept hurting myself on the vault because I was wild and took too many risks. I thought I was a mediocre athlete because I couldn't do a split. The fact I was the fastest girl in my school and a terrific basketball player didn't matter all that much because no one around me valued that until I got into middle school. That's what happens when we let other people's mirrors define who we are.

Oddly enough the researchers in the study concluded that both groups need to cut back on how much television they watch, which is old news, but they didn't see the other window of opportunity resting right there in the list of activities that African American girls like to do: church.

If they live in unsafe neighborhoods and attend schools that rarely listen to what they want in terms of physical activity, then why not go to the other place where they spend their leisure hours and, perhaps, the one place where they trust everyone around them and the space itself. My journey has brought me through the history of our sedentary culture and its physical and social consequences, but to reach this inner core of at-risk Americans I must go deeper to a spiritual stop that brings together both meanings of the word "grace."

I discovered something called Fitness Ministries, a trend that took firm hold in white Methodist churches in the U.S. in the 1980s. Pastors sold millions of copies of books like *Body By God*, and church-sponsored gyms like Lord's Gym, in Los Angeles, brought hundreds of thousands of parishioners to regular exercise for the first time in their lives. While some of the programs focused on weight loss, often to a neurotic and distorted degree, others included physical activity and talked less about fat as sinful and more about health as a celebration.

Several recent studies concluded that exercise programs run through churches have higher retention rates than secular recreational programs, which makes sense to me because they deal with *fear* and *lack* more directly. Even someone who lives in a housing project can find sanctuary in a city church. Even an immigrant working two low-wage jobs to make ends meet can make it to church on Sundays. Sufficient time in a safe place; a sense of community and trusted leaders.

I wanted to see a Fitness Ministry at work, which is how I came to be in the cool, dark, slanting open space of Saint Anthony's Catholic Church in Falls Church, Virginia. Hundreds of yards of silk white cloth hung across the ceiling in the shape of a cross. Two Hispanic workers, clearly fresh from some construction site, sat in the pews to my left. I was waiting for Georgine Redmond, the parish nurse and fitness minister of this congregation, which has 8,000 parishioners, most of them Hispanic.

Georgine herself is a short, stout middle-aged white woman with quick blue eyes. She spent most of her career working as an administrator at George Mason University, but eventually earned a doctorate in gerontology (health for the aged). After she retired from GMU, she "wanted to join the three threads: educational, physical, and spiritual" and began volunteering as the health nurse at St. Anthony's. Most of her work involves home visits to the elderly, counseling on how to navigate the healthcare system, and hospital visits.

As Georgine quickly makes clear to me, exercise did not top the list of healthcare concerns when parishioners filled out questionnaires. Seventy percent of them have no health insurance. Most have never been to a dentist. When they learn that they have high blood pressure or high blood sugar at one of the church-sponsored health fairs, there are few places they can go for follow-up tests and care. It's hard for them to really grasp that a better diet and more exercise could dramatically improve their overall health and could be their best answer. They go to a doctor or nurse to find a cure, not advice on preventive medicine.

The one thing they all agree on: Sunday is sacrosanct. They come by the thousands to the masses after their long work weeks. They walk across crazy Route 7 with their children in hand or they arrive by vanloads. At the 1:00 p.m. Sunday Spanish-language mass I attend at Saint Anthony's, people stand six deep in the aisles after the pews fill.

A guitarist plays some folk-like church music and a small chorus sings along in Spanish. The room fills with chatter, song, and huge families. Other than the priests on the altar, I am the only Caucasian person in the church. I could be in Mexico, El Salvador, or Columbia. I can see in their faces that they are home when they are here.

So the church provides a sense of community, safety, and leisure all at once, which makes it a very fertile place to try out new programs with populations that don't even have regular exercise on their radar screens. Georgine did precisely that when she started her "Walking With St. Paul" program, which asked parishioners to work in groups or as individuals to follow (in a symbolic sense) Apostle Paul's second and longest missionary journey (A.D. 50-51), a 2,800-mile trek from Syria through Macedonia and Greece.

She showed me the huge chart on a poster board in the church lobby. Laminated tags with names like Choir Walkers, Wannabees, Wisdom Walkers, and Ushers are pinned onto various points along a map of Paul's journey. The groups work out over the week, use pedometers to measure their distance, then tally their total. The Ushers in particular are really hoofing and are already almost "back" to Antioch.

"I knew I wanted to start a walking program, but that's not enough. I knew I needed a schtick to get people involved," Georgine says. She had heard about the St. Paul program at a conference, so she decided to try it out on her Hispanic congregation.

"At least half of the people in the program had never done any regular exercise before."

As we stare at the map, I think to myself, if she can get even 100 people who have never walked regularly before to find the time and energy in their week to move outside for leisure and health, that's amazing. When I think about all the obstacles that this particular Hispanic population faces—the lack of pedestrian-friendly walking areas, poverty, a poor diet, extra weight, significant health problems—I am humbled. In all my years as an athlete, I have never pulled off such a feat of discipline and commitment.

I flip through the Spanish-English packet Georgine pulled together as a handout. She lists all the potential health benefits from walking, including relieving stress, reducing cholesterol, lowering blood pressure, and strengthening bones. Then she makes "suggestions for walking in prayer."

Meditate on a passage from Scripture:

*Before you walk, choose a passage from the next few pages to think
and pray about. How does this verse impact your daily life?
Read Philippians 1. As you walk with Apostle Paul, think of
what he wrote to you and those he visited in Philippi.*

In Philippians, Paul writes of humility, thanksgiving, and deliverance. "We do all things through Christ who strengthens us." (Phil. 4:13)

That's the closest thing I find to advice on caring for our physical bodies in Philippians 1. Of course, people lived such labor-intensive lives 2,000 years ago that there was no need for weight-loss programs, fitness routines, or anything that artificial, so there's little talk of "exercise" per se in the Bible. Plenty of strong verbs fill the pages, however; people plant, harvest, steal, marry, and engage in all the stages of the average human life. As with any religious text, a person can find whatever they need in the Bible's pages.

In Corinthians, Paul does write, "Do you not know that your body is a temple of the Holy Spirit within you, which you have from God?" (1 Cor. 6:20)

The definitive authority on the history of the English language, the Oxford English Dictionary (OED), says the word *Holy* probably derives from an Old English word used prior to the rise of Christianity—*Hailo*—which means free from injury, whole, hale. Another derivative, *hailiz*, means health, happiness, and good luck. How fascinating that the third portion of the Holy Trinity, the portion that signifies God within us, is defined by a word related to *physical* health.

Of course the word *spirit* originally meant the animating or vital force in man and animals. The combination *Holy Spirit* didn't enter into regular use until as late as the 1500s. Either way this very spiritual term finds its roots in two words that point directly to physical well-being as *central* to an individual's spiritual well-being. To be filled with the Holy Spirit in the most literal sense, even for a person who follows no faith, is to be free from injury in all the vital aspects of the body.

Georgine tries to track down even one Latino walker in the Saint Paul program who will talk to me about their goals and motivations, but many of these people have a deep fear of giving their name to anyone. They might be here illegally or simply distrust anyone who wants personal information from them. I know I was able to reach the Hispanic women at the Family Place because I had Matilde Palmer with me. I have no such intermediary here and weeks go by with no success. I sense that I have introduced fear into a sacred contract between Georgine and her parishioners, which dismays me. I decide to back off and head to Mount Olive Baptist Church across town, an African American church that boasts one of the longest-running Fitness Ministry programs in the Capital area.

LaVaeda Coulter, a weight-lifting, hard-walking, smiling African American woman comes to her interview with two huge poster board charts in hand. As far back as 1998, LaVaeda pushed her pastor to incorporate exercise into the overall church program.

She admits, "People in the Baptist churches like to eat. We like to eat," she repeats for emphasis and with a forgiving laugh, as though visions of fried chicken are in her own head as she speaks. She could see firsthand every Sunday that her fellow parishioners suffered from diabetes, obesity, heart conditions, and more, and as a certified physical education instructor she decided to use movement to bring about change.

Unlike Georgine, who used Saint Paul for structure and motivation, LaVaeda relied on pure old-fashioned competition and challenged several other churches in the area to a walkathon. The rules: each congregation had three months to walk as many miles as possible. The group with the highest final total wins.

The numbers before me on one of the boards provide a detailed record of Mount Olive's successful charge to the top of the pedometer heap. The same strand of Scripture that Georgine cited in her pamphlet runs across the top: "We can do all things through Christ who strengthens us." (Phil. 4:3) I scan the mileage totals and see that LaVaeda herself logged 355 miles, and another ambitious walker pulled in more than 500. All told, the 170 or so participants achieved a group total of more than 19,000 miles.

"We had a slow start," LaVaeda confides, "but we came on in the end" (a polite way of saying they won).

I see gold stars next to certain names—probably people with exceptional totals. Even today, three years after the actual walking contest, LaVaeda points to the stars with real pride.

"You know, first I had to convince them they could walk. They'd say they can't walk, and I'd say, 'How'd you get here? You came up those stairs.' I'd put a pedometer on them and have them walk through their day so they could see for themselves how many steps they were taking," she says, her expressive brown eyes looking directly into mine as she speaks. I sense that LaVaeda will always savor this victory, always save the charts before me even when the glue begins to give and the numbers begin to fade because she harnessed something unique for her church—hope, vitality, and community spirit.

A woman named Freddie, wearing a Breast Cancer Walkathon T-shirt, enters the room where LaVaeda and I stand. She's here to pick up a book but can't help but join in the conversation about The Walk, which she participated in.

"We're thinking about challenging some of the churches in the District," she says. "We'd join with Zion," the other mighty Baptist congregation that was their biggest competitor in the last round.

I'm feeling good all around as I stand on the plush red-carpeted space just outside the main chapel. But then Freddie brings up kids. Lots of overweight, under-active African American kids, who literally fill the pews on Sunday to an alarming degree.

"When I was young we had all of that Presidential Fitness stuff and recess and gym. We're losing all of that. I can see it in the kids in this congregation." Both women are wide eyed with agreement and concern. We all discuss the lack of free play, the fear of public spaces, the car-oriented streets.

LaVaeda has placed all sorts of Christian-themed fitness materials on the bench next to me, including a Fitness Starter Kit, part of Lifeway's Christian Wellness Plan. Preaching about the body as the Holy Temple has become big business for a lot of people, something many critics view with contempt, because these programs often take the approach that fatness is sinful and the thin, white, Protestant model is the ideal.

But the idea that somehow at-risk populations might listen better about lifestyle-related problems if they hear it from a pastor or trusted fellow parishioner rather than in a school health class or from a doctor or even a television ad makes perfect sense. In the literature that LaVaeda handed out for her walking programs, I see no sign that she held up one particular model as an ideal. Instead she wrote in general of how "a fit child of God is a productive child of God." In her eyes, "Physical stewardship is an act of worship."

If churches stick to their mandate as safe havens—not places of profit or judgment—then Fitness Ministries could be the one best way to get people of any faith back into healthy movement patterns on a daily basis.

The American Nursing Association clearly saw the potential back in the 1990s when it officially recognized Health Ministry as a distinct subspecialty within the profession. Today the Health Ministry Association, a national organization, has thousands of members. Locally, near me in Virginia, the INOVA Congregational Health Partnership (CIP), a nonprofit hospital-based group, works with more than sixty churches in the area to develop Fitness Ministry programs.

"Church is the one place where there's a level of trust," Peggy Steen, who directs CIP, tells me. She works with a rainbow coalition of programs. I see binders in her office marked with black letters: KOREAN, HISPANIC, AFRICAN AMERICAN.

Steen, who has cropped sable hair and blue eyes that stare unblinking through her glasses, fell into the job after years of working around the world in health-related fields. The wife of a retired Foreign Service officer, Steen is fluent in Spanish, a huge selling point in this area. She doesn't say it outright, but it's clear that it's been slow going with the local church programs. Most of them don't like the idea of an outsider—even a well-intentioned one—swooping in with advice. She talks briefly about one twelve-week walking program she's helped start at a Hispanic church, but it's clear to me by the time I leave that CIP provides information, volunteers, and even a little money, but in the end, real success requires someone from within, like LaVaeda Coulter.

But LaVaeda herself is going to school and working full time. There are no fitness programs on the docket right now at Mount Olive, and over at Saint Anthony's, Georgine, who has done all her work over the last two years for free, wants and needs a salary. Both of these programs have huge, needy congregations, and yet even they struggle to sustain their Fitness Ministry agenda.

In the end, the pastors need to get on board. They need to see that the horrible physical decline of the most at-risk populations in America mirrors a spiritual decline. When I spoke with pastors like Father "Tuck" Grinnell at Saint Anthony's Catholic Church, they uniformly expressed concern, but they also seemed more comfortable discussing measurable things, like the number of blood tests taken at the church health fair, rather than the abstract—possible ways to alter the poor lifestyle habits of a large group of people. In the first instance, they must set up a nurse by a table, but in the second, they must motivate, guide, organize, and cajole. There's no debating which is the harder task.

At work and home we deal with the concrete everyday, but we go to church, to synagogue, to temple because we wish to touch the unseen within us and around us. If even houses of worship cannot nurture a stronger connection between physical and spiritual grace, then where can these at-risk populations find answers? To heal, they need safe havens. To change, they need understanding and education.

Once again, because it bears repeating as others before us have repeated it for more than two thousand years: "Do you not know that your body is a temple of the Holy Spirit within you, which you have from God?" (1 Cor. 6:20)

12

The Morality in Play

My bicycle accident and back surgery left me with a peculiar stiffness on my right side that starts in my hip and runs right up through the side of my face, which droops and twitches when I tire. Exercise and physical therapy have done little to remedy the problem. People often interpret my stiffness as social coolness, which made me curious about the connection between kinesthetic intelligence and declining civility in American society.

Most educators embrace Howard Gardner's idea of multiple intelligences, such as mathematical, musical, bodily, and interpersonal. No one is exceptional in all areas. I know personally my mathematical intelligence is, at best, about average, for example, but my physical acumen has always been sharp, even when I was very young. I come from a long line of athletes on both sides of my family and also developed my innate talents by moving around for hours at a time for decades on end.

I actually had an opportunity to test what Gardner calls my bodily-kinesthetic intelligence while working as an English teacher at a technical high school in Virginia. The man in charge of shop challenged me to take some sort of hand/eye test that involved moving objects around rapidly to their correct slots. My hands moved faster than my mind as I slipped round things into round holds and small widgets into small widget spaces. He was so stunned at the accuracy and speed of my results, he asked me to do it again. I improved. No one had ever come close to my total score, he said.

I tell this tale not to brag, but to showcase how I managed to hyper-develop my physical self through a combination of inherited ability and training. Clearly I lacked such natural talents in math, and certainly didn't apply myself to my training. End result: a D in Algebra II my junior year in high school.

I heard again and again what would happen to me if I didn't improve my math scores: lousy SATs, poor college choices, no chance for a career in the sciences. But I don't ever remember anyone ever telling me or anyone else I knew about the long-term consequences of low body awareness. I excelled as an athlete so I never gave it much thought until I lost my ability to move freely after my back accident. Suddenly I found myself feeling awkward in certain social situations because I *had* to stand every thirty minutes or so. I *had* to turn to my right very stiffly. My reduced physical mobility not only impaired my social grace, but also devastated my social life. I could no longer do team sports. I could no longer take long airplane rides for vacation trips, sit in restaurants for two-hour dinner parties, or even attend church.

Right around the time I was struggling with all of this, I began work on a book on the Wright brothers for National Geographic as part of a celebration of the Centennial of Flight in 2003. Engineers and aviation buffs all across the country wanted to build and fly a replica of the original Wright *Flyer*, a blend of canvas and wood that took off from the sands of North Carolina's Outer Banks on December 17, 1903, and ushered in the world of human flight. The most serious groups looked at the brothers' original journals and the original airplane, which now hangs in the foyer of the Smithsonian's National Air and Space Museum in Washington, D.C. Several people built some very handsome replicas, but no one—*no one*—managed to craft *and* fly a reproduction of the original *Flyer*.

I mention this because the brothers themselves, two bicycle shop owners from Ohio, solved one of the great mysteries of the natural world because they *physically* engaged in every inch of their famous machine. The first prototypes required the two men to develop a finely tuned sense of their own center of gravity as they sat in their glider-like contraptions. After a few hair-raising nosedives, they realized they needed to figure out a way to control their flying machine while in the air—something (amazingly enough) most previous researchers hadn't spent much time thinking about. They devised a cradle for their hips that had wires attached to the wings, which they could then tilt up or down, depending on the needs of the moment. They had to work the rudder with their hand via a stick and shift their hips left and right in the cradle to keep the wings in line.

Now to give contemporary engineers some slack, the *Flyer* was notoriously squirrelly and would nosedive without warning. The fact the Wright brothers survived their own experiments is definitely one of the most amazing athletic feats (not just scientific) of all time. It made sense to add a few modern touches to insure a safe landing during Centennial of Flight demonstrations around the country.

But I'm convinced that today's pilots and engineers also failed because they simply lacked the Wright brothers' superb physical intelligence. Most pilots today spend an amazing amount of their training time in front of screens where they "fly" using a simulator. Most never physically handle a rudder and certainly do not use their body to shift the angle of the aileron (the famous tilting wing). At the Smithsonian, just down the hallway from the original *Flyer*, visitors can "fly" an airplane, again while sitting in a chair and looking at a screen. The disconnect between what these "pilots" do and what their bodies sense—very little, since they just sit and engage few muscle groups—leaves them in a world almost completely dominated by their mind. And while the problem of flight was certainly an intellectual Mount Everest, it was also a *physical* problem.

Of course my sense that American society has seen a dramatic collective decline in its overall physical intelligence quotient was just a hunch, a conclusion I'd reached based on my own experiences. So none of the Centennial celebrants could replicate what the Wright brothers had done; well, no one had pulled it off for hundreds of years before the two men showed up either.

To explore my theory I sought out some experts at the Laban/Bartenieff Institute of Movement headquartered in New York City, which specializes in how people flow through space. First conceived by Rudolf Laban, a Hungarian immigrant who is known as the father of European modern dance, the Laban

Method applies precise terms to describe things, such as the difference between punching someone in the face and reaching for a glass. The two actions are quite similar, but differ in their speed and intent. The "Bartenieff" portion of the institute comes from one of Laban's original students in the 1950s, Irmgard Bartenieff, who broke Laban's broad concepts down into even more precise forms of measurements, including things like Core Support, Spatial Intent, and Dynamic Alignment. By quantifying the differences in physical action, the teachers felt they could show others how to replicate the action and provide guidelines for movement, especially for professional actors, politicians, and dancers.

Karen Bradley, current chair of the institute, splits her time between New York City and Washington, D.C., where she lives in a row house behind Capitol Hill. I made my way over there on an August afternoon to hear her thoughts on body language in the U.S. today.

While standing on her stoop, I note the molding around the high windows and the red front door. When she actually opens the door, I am looking up and slightly to my left. I'm certain she sees a story in that action—perhaps shyness—since she's an expert at reading faces and other mannerisms.

She's been hired to analyze the facial expressions of presidential candidates and even President George W. Bush during his State of the Union Address. *New Yorker* magazine writer Malcolm Gladwell interviewed her for a profile he did on the renowned dog handler Cesar Millan (host of "Dog Whisperer" on the National Geographic television channel). She analyzed Millan's body movements for evidence of why even the most violent dogs react positively to him. She looked at where he placed his hands, how he squatted on his hips and when. She described his various movements as "phases" and used words like "impactive" and "explosive."

I shake her hand and make sure to make direct eye contact. She's small, about five feet, in her fifties, fair of face with wire-rimmed glasses. She does not move like a dancer or athlete; more like a regular neighborhood walker. But her green-hazel eyes are wide, expressive, and really engage with me when I speak to her. She feels very *present* when she talks.

She agrees that "Today, kids have an issue with embodiment. They are not masters of time and space anymore. They don't do enough diverse activity.

They might be good at one thing, but the rest of the time they're sitting down in front of the TV or at their computers." The end result: "They don't see their own impact on the world. They don't see consequences well. They think, because of all of the TV and movies that they watch, 'I can erase it and start over again.'"

I think about the way people move around me in the grocery store or in a crowded subway station. Many of them, and not just kids, are listening to music through headsets or talking on a cell phone. All the people they know and call every day, all the things they have hanging over them at work and at home, can now come with them wherever they are thanks to gadgets like a BlackBerry. They have an invisible box that they carry around with them whenever they move. I can bump into that box (or that box bumps into me), and they register the interruption as a flicker and then retreat to their "living room" again. As Dr. Bradley talks, I recall a couple I saw sitting in a restaurant recently. As soon as they sat down, the man whipped out his cell phone and began talking to someone. His head tipped away from the woman and into the receiver. The couple's hands touched, but their upper torsos were directed away from each other.

Technology has really skewed our relationship with the four areas that the Laban Movement focuses on: space, time, weight, and flow. I notice that when Dr. Bradley's phone rings, she does not answer it or take her eyes off my face. When her son comes through the front door, she acknowledges him with her voice, but I remain her focus. I am her guest, and I never lose that feeling the entire time I'm in her house.

"Each of us has a physical bubble and if we can master that, well, that's a huge step toward creativity and stability," she says.

To help people live in the *now* in time and space, she teaches them how to breathe.

"Inhalation breath is inspirational and exhalation is expressive. Neither phase is passive. What we need to be doing is walking out and being inspired by the world and giving our own response to it. We would all be more productive, relaxed, and honest."

Without empathy, without body awareness, without focused attention on the person at hand, it's difficult to sustain a civil self.

Each person has their own special way of recuperating from their day. As Dr. Bradley points out, most Americans choose to sit in front of a television or computer screen, but that's probably not the right recuperative state for most of us.

"People don't even explore these things anymore," she says, adjusting her glasses slightly for emphasis. She often uses music in her programs, especially with disturbed kids, because it provides rhythm and sequence. "Rhythm is mastery of time, it's organizing, and kids without sequencing in their lives can use it to help them feel more stable." But, she adds, the recuperative state could just as easily be kneading bread or knitting. The point is people don't try to figure that out for themselves anymore; they just passively give in to the media stimulation around them.

She walks me to the door. We shake hands and again establish excellent eye contact.

As I move toward my car, I think about my posture, the pace of my steps, the angle of my shoulders. I think about the message my physical self gives to the world.

Dr. Bradley herself insists that body intelligence is the *first* intelligence because "we're born to physically interact immediately."

But we've developed a culture that has forgotten how to center the physical self. Today so much movement is concentrated in the hands as we work remotes and keyboards. The play of the rest of the body becomes irrelevant. While shopping in the tight spaces of my local Whole Foods, I've seen people listening to iPods reach for something in the produce section and their movement definitely feels more like a punch in the face than reaching for a glass.

Problems with civility rarely rise above more than an irritation; but, according to neurologist Dr. Antonio Damasio, author of *Descartes' Error: Emotion, Reason, and the Human Brain,* and director of the Brain and Creativity Institute at the University of California, sitting in front of a screen all day watching violent or emotionally disturbing images does more than erode bodily awareness; it impairs people's *moral* judgment. The cognitive part of the brain, which deals with things like remembering names and problem solving, can pick up the pace as it circles through the day like a good miler with a kick, but the *emotional* part of the brain requires more complex steps to operate. When you read your boss's face to see if she's pleased or displeased with your work, you must tap into something that Damasio calls somatic markers—basically a memory bank of appropriate behaviors and patterns. That takes time; there's no rushing the process.

"We really have two systems that are totally integrated and work perfectly well with each other but are very different in their time constraints," he explained in a *Discover* magazine interview. "One is the emotional system, which is the basic regulatory system that works very slowly, with timescales of a second or more. Then you have the cognitive system, which is much faster because of the way it's wired."

In thirty minutes of television, thousands of images flash on the screen that encourage or even demand an emotional response: someone gets shot; a cop finds a young woman's bloody body spread across a bedroom floor; scenes of real children wounded in Iraq appear on the evening news. According to Damasio, the human brain can follow the quick-paced shift in topics, but it cannot generate a fully formed response to so much complex emotional stimuli in such a short amount of time.

Psychologists who studied the aftermath of 9/11 found that people who watched re-runs of the terrorists hitting the World Trade Center towers in New York again and again were far more apt to have post-traumatic stress disorder. Children in particular often responded on a deep emotional level *each* time they saw the footage replayed. They had trouble comprehending that the violence was out there and had already happened. Adults, who can handle more complex notions of space and time, coped more effectively, but only because their minds became numb to the violence.

I know the first time I watched footage of the airplanes striking the towers, a tremendous anxiety swept through me like an electrically charged hand and left me overwhelmed with sadness and confusion. Now I sense the residual of those feelings whenever I see the same images, but not their full vigor.

This desensitizing process is essential for human's emotional well-being, but when applied to a media-saturated environment where people watch four to five hours of television or DVDs a day, a large percentage of which contain violent imagery, abusive emotional situations, and sexually charged dramatic scenes, then people run the risk of emotionally disengaging from most of what they see, just so they can handle it.

"The image of an event or a person can appear in a flash," Dr. Damasio said in the same interview, "but it takes seconds to make an emotional marking. So it stands to reason that we're going to have fewer and fewer chances to have appropriate somatic markers, which means we're going to have more and more events—particularly in the earlier years—that go by without the emotional grounding, which means that you could potentially be ethically less grounded. You'd be in an emotionally neutral world."

If Damasio is correct, then we have a culture that encourages children to develop an emotionally muted response to the narratives—real and unreal—playing out around them. While the direct link between watching violence on a screen and actually committing more violence remains inconclusive, many studies show that people who watch more TV (of any type) have a much higher tolerance for violence in everyday life. Mass media overloads Americans' emotional circuits on a daily basis and possibly impacts our moral center on a *biological* level, especially among young viewers. So I may have made the ultimate parental miscue by forcing my daughter into behaviors that left her socially isolated, but that doesn't change the fact that her generation's tendency to turn to screens rather than sunny skies and spontaneous outdoor activities for release and relaxation is impacting not only their long-term physical health—we hear lots about that—but also their social and moral intelligence, which almost no one talks about, especially not the mainstream media.

What the press does focus on a lot is the financial bang imposed by poor lifestyle habits: 70 to 80 percent of the healthcare costs (about two trillion a year) in this country spring from our sedentary habits and crummy food choices. The average family today pays almost $11,000 a year for health coverage, a devastating chunk of the family and employer cash flow. We incur such personal and financial costs, in part, because of a collective lapse of will power among individuals, employers, and every level of government, which makes it a moral issue, since some of what's wrong arises from choices under our control.

To fully see all of the players involved, imagine an overweight diabetic who doesn't exercise and has an inconsistent diet. He works for a small employer whose overall health-insurance premiums go up because of the diabetic's expensive care. The other employees get angry when they learn they must pay an additional $15 a month for the insurance hike. Meanwhile the diabetic *does* want to improve, but can't walk or bike to work because of unsafe roads, time, and distance. There's no place to work out on site. He brings his own food most days, but when he forgets, the only options locally are the vending machines and a McDonald's down the street.

Of course the diabetic is responsible for his own lifestyle choices, but at every turn his employer and society make those bad choices almost inevitable. Fortunately, all of the players in this hypothetical scenario have begun to acknowledge their role in the country's collective lifestyle crisis. According to a survey conducted by the *Wall Street Journal* in 2006, more than half of Americans feel it would be fair to make people with unhealthy lifestyles pay higher insurance premiums. Three years ago that figure was just 35 percent.

The same year, in West Virginia, the state launched a pilot Medicaid program, which strives to be more proactive about helping people make better lifestyle choices. Participants, who get involved in classes and activities that provide guidance on diet, smoking, exercise, and other wellness topics, earn credits that can then be used for things such as a free membership in a local sports club.

Of course the problem with such carrots is they smack of blackmail. As Dr. Robert Steinbrook asked in his analysis of the West Virginia program, "Imposing Personal Responsibility for Health," in the *New England Journal of Medicine*: "Which well-meaning measures to promote responsible behavior actually make a difference and which are primarily coercive and potentially counterproductive?"

While I agree with Dr Steinbrook's skepticism and know that educational programs alone will not bring about lasting changes in behavior, I am heartened by the effort and the intent of the West Virginia plan. At least it tries to make people more accountable, and it acknowledges that government and employers trying similar reward programs must play some role because they, too, are part of the problem.

Effective solutions seem to involve social pressure and support. The most astounding study of the power of peer pressure that I found in my research involved 333 patients recovering from open-heart surgery. The insurance company, Mutual of Omaha, wanted to know why *90 percent* of them returned to the lifestyle habits that led to their heart problems in the first place, even though the surgery itself is incredibly traumatic and involves sawing open a patient's chest, among other intrusions. Why would anyone do anything that might cause them to repeat the experience?

To find out, Dr. Dean Ornish, professor of medicine at the University of California, in San Francisco, and his team of researchers took the patients through a twice-weekly group support session and provided instruction in yoga, meditation, and aerobic exercise. The program lasted only a year, but after three years, 77 percent of the patients had stuck with the lifestyle changes and avoided surgery altogether. Mutual of Omaha saved $30,000 a patient despite footing the bill for the yearlong program.

Dr. Ornish's team found that neither crisis nor fear nor facts alone could bring about lasting change. Treatment must first focus on that emotional center that Dr. Damasio has written so much about. The team enhanced the patients' sense of community by working in group sessions and talked about their recovery in terms of finding joy rather than avoiding death. Dr. Ornish insisted on aggressive changes across the board in diet, exercise, and attitude rather than incremental shifts, probably the most important breakthrough of all. People change patterns sooner and stick with it longer if the change is extreme.

For now, despite such studies, Americans live in a world of incremental solutions. The gaming industry, for example, doesn't really want you to let go of that console, but it knows it must also appease the sedentary-police like me. Nintendo's low-cost, user-friendly Wii is the ideal half-answer—the very thing Dr. Ornish claims will not work in the long haul—but has certainly silenced a lot of critics in the short term. Players use small white remotes to "play" tennis, baseball, bowl, or even to box against either the machine itself or a real live opponent, who also uses a remote to make things happen on the screen. Kids can get so energetic swinging at virtual balls that remotes often go flying. (Nintendo had to install much sturdier straps on the remotes after the Wii first came out.)

When this interactive game hit stores, it outsold the much fancier (and expensive) Sony PlayStation3 and Microsoft Xbox 360; everyone from eight-year-old boys to seniors at retirement homes were punching, rolling, and swinging with their Wiis. A whole new crowd of Americans got introduced to the joys of gaming.

I bought one for my daughter. After all, my more aggressive approach of severe restrictions on hours and access to all this media had backfired.

The first few times we played tennis or boxed, we did break a sweat, but we quickly figured out how to move a lot less and accomplish a lot more with the remotes. At this point, my daughter can beat me sitting down, if she feels like it.

In the end the Wii, and other games like it, just reinforces a screen-based worldview that will never lead to the more dramatic lifestyle changes Americans need to make to match the success of the patients in Dr. Ornish's study. We are like the 90 percent of heart surgery patients who return home, do some physical therapy exercises while watching a movie, but soon resort to simply eating in front of the screen instead. We find the media easier than the yoga or the walking, and since we are operating in isolation and the collective social pressure actually pushes us closer to the screen, we soon find ourselves back on the surgeon's table under the saw. Somehow we manage to be shocked—yes, shocked—to be there again.

In a recent *Wired* magazine special *Home* edition, the editors profiled what they thought the American home would look like in 2010. They predicted that most people would have a central media server that would provide them everything everywhere in their home, from movies, music, television, Internet access, and even dim lights upon request. "Never Leave Couch Again," declared one upbeat headline.

The article opens with a doctored photograph of a lean young woman gracefully holding a LCD touch screen. The person in that picture in the real future will be neither thin nor physically elegant if Americans follow where *Wired* magazine, or even the Wii for that matter, expects them to go.

I began this book to chronicle my own efforts to rebuild my broken body and to see what we could do to rebuild the collective American body. While in recovery, I knew I would miss the heavy sweats of intense exercise and the camaraderie of pickup basketball games. I knew I would have to alter my social life and avoid lengthy dinners in restaurants and even jobs that required extensive deskwork.

But I did not anticipate the guilt. As the tone in my muscles faded, I felt inferior. When I put on a few pounds around my waist, I felt unattractive. When I started eating too many sweets and drinking coffee regularly to help alleviate some of my depression, I felt weak.

The structure of American society imposes the same sort of restrictions on the collective public as my ruptured disks. It sets parameters that make if very difficult to maneuver. The resulting emotional stress often presses people to seek out unhealthy forms of relief, including, in my case, poorer eating and depression. It's dispiriting to be constantly placed in a situation where you feel morally weak, which is how I feel when my will power falters.

If I had a group, like Dr. Ornish's group, to go to three times a week that gave me encouragement and advice and a physical routine implemented by me and others around me, my recovery would have been so much faster. Instead, I felt I had to hide the fact I had to work standing up, that I was no longer the athlete I once was, and that I felt horribly isolated in my new reduced situation.

My doctor bluntly told me I had about a 90 percent chance of returning to his surgery table in two to three years for a "tune up," because of weight gain and a tendency to revert to old habits, such as too much sitting all day. He sent me to a physical therapist for a few weeks, but then that was it; I was home alone faced with a 95 percent reduction in my exercise time and a job as a writer and editor that required extensive sitting. I never received any social support from a group of fellow back surgery patients or any dietary advice as a newcomer to the calorie-counting club.

My great love for vigor, the outdoors, and my strong sense of personal responsibility for my own health, ultimately motivated me to stick with a self-created program of swimming, physical therapy, walking, and a special ratio of standing and sitting throughout my day that allowed me to regain my physical self. It's what I knew and lived as a child on a physical and moral level that saved me—not my doctor, or my community, or my employer. Of course, for more people to succeed where I almost failed, these three groups must get more involved.

It's downright terrifying to know that if had grown up in the future envisioned by *Wired* magazine, I would have never recovered from my accident, never returned to exercise for hours every week, never conquered my depression. I would have returned to the surgeon's table, but not my own life as I wanted to live it.

And whose fault would that be?

13

This Is Your Brain on Exercise

When I don't move enough, I get depressed. A smothering hand reaches into my mind and makes it difficult for me to focus and engage with others socially, even my own family. I had some bouts in the past, but the accident, back surgery, and resulting immobility pressed that proverbial hand into my mind longer and harder than I could ever remember. I knew if I did not get back to some sort of regular physical activity, I could sink into a black hole I might never get out of.

While studying the impact that exercise has on the brain, I found that many scientists believe that depression is a form of hibernation, a deliberate attempt at no movement because regular movement means an active life; and if things are not going well, you naturally want to withdraw into some sort of holding pattern. One writer called it a "brain lock," which was the closest I've come to finding a phrase that describes what my mind felt like during my years of limited mobility. (The reverse, of course, is my life when I am fit and active: bursting with mental and physical energy and able to survive easily on five or six hours of sleep a day. I like to think of this animated state as "brain open.")

On some level, I suspect that the 65 percent of Americans who do not exercise several days a week suffer from symptoms associated with a hibernating brain; but while some research proves my hypothesis, no expert I interviewed would flatly state that the majority of Americans are in some sort of collective depressed state. I do know that our brains evolved based on the movement patterns of hunter-gatherers, and something as simple as shooting a basketball taps into many sections of the brain. The cerebellum, for example, maintains balance, regulates muscle tone and coordination, but portions of the cerebral cortex actually signal when a muscle should become active.

All you have to do is look inside the womb at a developing embryo to see the incredible link between physical movement and brain development and health. A fetus first moves as early as six weeks, though most women don't actually feel anything until about the tenth week. Doctors call this sensation "quickening," a word that has a splendid poetic quality because it hints at an awakening of sorts, a rush forward toward full life. By five months a fetus can bring her thumb to her mouth.

"Given how neural activity critically shapes developing dendrites and synapses, this steady stream of fetal movement is probably the single most important form of stimulation a fetus brain receives," Dr. Lize Eliot, a professor of neuroscience at the Chicago Medical School, writes in *What's Going On in There? How the Brain and Mind Develop in the First Five Years of Life.* By the end of the first trimester, a fetus can hiccup, stretch, yawn, suck, swallow, grasp, and probably even twinkle its toes.

Once born, of course, a baby's success becomes measured by yet other physical milestones: holding her head up, rolling over, sitting up, taking her first step. It's clear to even a new parent that these physical milestones correspond on a fundamental level with proper brain development and reflect not just a healthy body, but also a healthy mind capable of reaching, yearning, grabbing, and learning.

But somewhere around age three or so, parents start focusing more on whether or not their child can recognize numbers or letters or, better yet, read by kindergarten. The milestones seem largely intellectually, and we tend to divorce what's happening in children's physical lives from what happens on a biological level in their brains. The gap becomes even more pronounced with each passing decade until adults assume almost no connection between their physical activity patterns and competency, and their mental acuity.

While working on this chapter, I consistently came across newspaper and magazine stories that encouraged elderly people to sharpen their brains with mental exercises, such as crossword puzzles. They plug products like Nintendo's *Brain Age 2*, a memory game involving simple math, or *MindFit*, which includes a personalized training regimen of mental exercises. One *New York Times* article even went so far as to lament that Americans spent only $225 million a year on so-called neurosoftware, but $16 billion a year on health-club memberships, as though physical activity had little to contribute to brain health.

Well, ditch the crossword puzzles and start walking because the most recent research shows that exercise is better than anything else you can do for your brain. As Dr. John Ratey states in his book, *Spark: The Revolutionary New Science of Exercise and the Brain*, physical activity is like Miracle-Gro for the mind, especially for those over fifty, and helps relieve anxiety and depression and improves mental focus. One study of 5,000 elderly people found that regular exercisers were *50 percent* less likely to develop any form of dementia.

Starting at age forty, most of us lose as much as 5 percent of our brain volume every decade; the decline accelerates once we hit seventy. Reading, complex problem solving, and similar mental gymnastics are excellent for sustaining active neurons (okay, so keep the puzzles), but *only* exercise can create *new* neurons and slow the overall decline in brain volume.

When I look at how fetuses evolve in the womb, it seems obvious that physical motion would lie at the root of new neuron development, but until the 1990s, scientists believed that we were born with all the neurons we would ever have and the adult brain could not create new ones. If someone injured a portion of his brain in an accident, for example, other areas of the brain might compensate and take on some of the tasks of the damaged area, but the lost neurons were lost forever and no new ones would spring up in their place.

In many key ways this theory is correct. In most areas of a newborn's brain, she has as many neurons as she'll ever have. Each of those neurons sprouts a root system called dendrites, which receives input from other neurons, and a trunk, or axon, which branches out to relay information to the next neuron in the circuit. When an impulse reaches the end of an axon, it must cross a gap, the synapse, in order to transmit to the next neuron in the circuit (a chemical messenger helps traverse the divide). The brain produces millions more neurons than it uses, and mainly only keeps those snatched up to form synapses, which are essentially communication points between two cells. Each time a child tries to learn a new letter, for example, she taps into neurons to form a synapse. In the first year of life, a child's cerebral cortex triples in thickness as a result of all of the branches (or dendrites) and synapses forming. Essentially, neurons start out as simple saplings, but a combination of genetics and a rich external environment builds them into strong, multiple-tiered trees.

But if we go back to our adult accident victim, who has a far less plastic brain than a newborn, there's no chance to triple the thickness of a damaged cerebral cortex or to replace the neurons lost from that portion of the brain. The faulty assumption scientists have made, however, is that the adult brain can *never* develop new neurons anywhere, which is not true.

In the 1990s, Dr. Fred Gage and several of his postdoctoral students at the Salk Institute in California, completed experiments that showed that physical exercise generated new neurons in adult brains of all ages in the hippocampus, an area of the mind that allows us to recall memories and link ideas. As is often the case, they began with mice, which they divided into two groups: those exposed just to an exercise wheel and those exposed to little exercise, but a more mentally challenging environment. Using a chemical marker that tracks the proliferation of cancer cells in patients, they tracked the proliferation of neurons in the mice's brains and found that the exercisers had *five* times more new cell development in their hippocampus area than the other group.

These startling findings convinced Dr. Gage to pursue this line of study with human brains, so they gathered tissue from adult humans of varying ages, and in 1998, became the first to publish a paper that officially proved that the adult brain does create new neurons, a process called neurogenesis, but *only* through exercise. A follow-up study in 2007 showed that the greater the level of exercise, the higher the level of neurogenesis.

I found Dr. Gage's work so enthralling and complex that I decided to track him down in California to talk with him in person about the more subtle aspects of his findings and where he thinks it could all lead. It felt so empowering to take this final step to complete this book because I had fully regained my own mental and physical health and, unlike my first trip to the Active Living Research Conference three years earlier, I could now fly to California with ease.

My methodical rehabilitation routine over more than five years, including a lot of work in the water, had allowed me to regain about 90 percent of my former mobility; I was free to move about the country.

Cyclists stream down Route 5 between my hotel and the Salk Institute in numbers that I'd never find on the East Coast in a major city. The broad bike lanes and sunny weather create a synergy that encourages all types to move on two wheels instead of four and a combustion engine. At the Salk Institute itself, I spy racks packed with bicycles and even a surfboard in a corner.

In the 1960s, Dr. Jonas Salk, who created the vaccine for polio, among other remarkable accomplishments, commissioned the architect Louis Kahn to create a laboratory center that would be "worthy of a visit by Pablo Picasso." The end result is one of the most unusual spaces I've ever walked through, with walls of solid concrete rising at sharp vertical angles and jutting out like wedges into a courtyard of blinding whiteness and flat lines. The Pacific Ocean meets the equally flat skyline in the distance, a visual effect that combines with the angular building to create a space that makes me feel as though I'm standing in the middle of some mathematical equation on a white board. This is clearly a scientist's idea of a nurturing space, but it must work because world-class scientists like Dr. Gage continue to come here to conduct their research.

Gage is a tall, trim, tan man with a sandy mustache and round wire-rimmed glasses. He has a boyish energy about him that makes him quite approachable, even though in conversation it's clear that his mind is working at a clip that makes me feel as though I'm thinking in slow motion. I watch his hands flick here and there as they play the part of neurons and synapses.

He summarizes the famous mice experiment for me but then adds another fascinating layer.

"It turned out that the enrichment did not have much of an impact on the proliferation, but increased the survival of those cells that were recently born. Normally a brain generates cells [neurons are just one type of cell in the brain] all of the time but about 50 percent of them die unless you actively engage them in some complexity; if you do that, then a greater percentage of them survive. If you combine physical activity with engagement of complexity you get an increase of cells and an increase of their survival. So they work together."

When I look at his face as he explains these things, I see the hazel eyes of a man in the thick of the creative process, alive with ideas and hope for the great potential of his life work. He seems to be almost laughing with a sort of joy that radiates even in his small office space, which he's plastered with framed covers from journals he's published in, like *Science* and *Nature,* as well as some playful posters and cartoons.

Of course this is very serious work that could have very positive implications for people with Parkinson's, Alzheimer's or other diseases that result from impaired neurons. If they can isolate the process and replicate it somehow, then they have the potential to help all sorts of people with neurological problems. A white board, covered with equations and the warning DO NOT ERASE, hangs on the wall behind me.

But Dr. Gage and I both agree that it's equally interesting to ponder the implications for the average person. What does it mean that most Americans don't move enough and deprive their brains of neuron-generating activities in the hippocampus, which helps us remember things and to place things in context, among other subtle but vital thinking skills? Normally when scientists talk about movement and the brain they focus on the basal ganglia, cerebellum, and brain stem, which govern most of the steps required for those bikers to zip up Route 5, for example. But Dr. Gage's work shows that exercise also has profound implications for our intellectual development and the mind/body split is an artificial divide.

"People have choices. If you choose to do a certain type of behavior or choose to not do a certain type of behavior, it's going to feedback into your brain and your brain will then behave in accordance with the choices you made. You ask why do people persist in not being physically active [despite being told how important it is to their health]? Well, if you're not physically active and have no history of it, your brain is changing to adapt to that lifestyle. . . . You must first change your behavior patterns, which will change your brain, which will allow you to do exercise in a more regular way. But it isn't something that's going to happen tomorrow. It is something that you will have to actively, deliberately engage in."

I think I just heard him tell me that by not exercising a person actually impairs their brain on some level so that it can't take up physical activity easily again without a very deliberate plan of action. For more than fifty years, Americans have heard how important regular exercise is to their general health, but an intractable percentage—65 percent—fail to alter their behavior; finally, someone who has some scientific answer for why simply hearing what's good for us isn't enough.

"So a six-week exercise class isn't going to undo a decade of inactivity and it's not just about will power?" I ask.

"It's not. Absolutely not," he replies.

I conjecture to myself that if I look at this equation in reverse, my brain got used to at least an hour of moderate to vigorous exercise five to six days a week for decades; when I had to withdraw from that pattern, I sent my neurogenesis process, among other things, into complete disarray. People who suffer from severe depression often have a smaller hippocampus. Based on Dr. Gage's findings, I was literally shrinking my own hippocampus with my forced inactivity.

Of course, as soon as I was able, I jumped at the chance to get moving again. It was difficult to work through the muscle weakness and sense of lethargy, but as an experienced athlete I knew all the gains I could make and what it would mean to my life, so I tackled the swimming and physical therapy with positive energy. My attitude turns out to have been as important as my action.

In an experiment conducted by one of Dr. Gage's graduate students, they found that mice *forced* to exercise on a moving treadmill did not generate any new neurons while those that voluntarily ran on a running wheel over the same distance did.

"The dark side of stress is that it represses neurogenesis," he explains. So if we drag people to exercise they won't reap the same benefits as those who go eagerly and willingly.

"They need to make it as positive an experience as possible. They don't need to do a lot. They can work their way up to different levels," Gage says. Personally, he plays squash, though he also walks, runs, and generally likes all forms of activity. He had a frightening car accident in college that forced him to undergo a lot of physical therapy and taught him to appreciate his body. Of course his own groundbreaking research on the brain and physical activity is probably all the inspiration he needs. The doctor takes his own medicine.

As I leave his office, I look out toward the Pacific, across the wide, flat expanse of concrete and white light, and feel as though I've just found something of great importance to me. My conversations with Dr. Gage armed me with new information about depression, the limits of will power, the crucial link between movement and brain health, and so much more. It's one thing to have an intuitive sense about something, like feeling that regular exercise is crucial to my mental balance, but it's another to have someone tell you that they're proving these connections on a cellular level. It's not just in my head, or, rather, it is—not as a loose idea, but as a provable physical phenomena.

I must use my hippocampus to reconstruct the interview with Dr. Gage. I see his tan face, a memory now as I type, and I recall strands of the conversation. I prod my memory with notes and a taped transcript, but some of the richest part of the interview came from personal observations that I must conjure up purely out of my own mind. Why would our adult brains evolve so that only this part would receive the benefits of neurogenesis generated by physical activity?

"We spend a lot of time thinking about, 'Why this brain structure?' which is so crucial for both emotions and learning and memory," Dr. Gage told me. "It's a new question, and we have a very discrete theory about it."

A very simplified version would go something like this: the hippocampus helps us discern between similar events. For example, Dr. Gage looks a lot like Dr. Steve Holen from the hunter-gatherer site I visited in Kansas, but I have no problem distinguishing between the two interview experiences. The same area of the brain also allows us to apply what we've learned from a given situation to a new, albeit, similar situation. The brain tries very hard to keep things separate, but there are times when we need to integrate memories and ideas. The hippocampus helps with both functions, and the new cells generated by neurogenesis, which tend to be highly excitable, may be crucial to the subtler job of integrating related memories and emotions.

In my mind I hypothesize that perhaps nature made allowances for physically robust hunter-gatherers, who could still remain active into their forties, by offsetting the natural decline of neurons as we age with new neurons in the hippocampus, where they generate a form of wisdom. Continued mobility indicates continued contributions; sharper memories and connections mean more intellectual currency to offer the group.

I actually threw the word "wisdom" out there, but Gage didn't pick up on it with any enthusiasm. Instead he gave me an example of sitting down to a particular Christmas dinner. Now I can put myself back at that Christmas dinner and that in turn may get me thinking about other Christmas dinners and now, perhaps, whenever I think of that first Christmas dinner, I'll also remember Dr. Gage telling me this story.

"How the heck do you link all of those things?" he asked me, knowing full well that the answer probably lies somewhere in his lab.

Now, if you recall a memory, like the Christmas dinner, but can't recall any other related things, then what?

"You're depressed," he claimed, then talked about Iraqi children traumatized by the war, who had experienced precisely that problem. The stress chopped their neurogenesis way down (another marker of depression), which in turn impaired not only their memory, but also their ability to make associations.

The violence deprives them of neighborhoods, proper schooling, normal social lives, and, it appears, even of memories.

I brought our conversation back to depression after this exchange and asked him my million-dollar question: Is America's sedentary majority living in some sort of depressed state because of the lack of neurogenesis in their brains?

"Hmm." He literally hmmmed. He looked at me as though he might say "yes," but clearly the scientific evidence doesn't yet point to such a direct link. "I wouldn't say it's that causal." We discuss my depression following my back surgery, and he wondered out loud: "Is it the loss of neurogenesis that causes depression or does the lack of plasticity set up a framework where things that you would normally adapt to, you are not able to adapt to any longer?"

He does think neurogenesis generated by physical activity creates a "neurological buffer" that probably helps people deal with difficult things more readily. Of course he's looking for specific evidence at the molecular level that can be repeated again and again in a lab, so he's far more cautious than a reporter like me about making blanket statements. I find "buffer" a bit tame as words go when I consider all that I gain from exercise in my life, but I know he agrees that movement impacts the mind on many positive levels, and neurogenesis is just one measure of that.

As he walked me to the door, Dr. Gage told me that he'd visited His Holiness the 14th Dalai Lama of Tibet, and studied the brain patterns of the monks, who, thanks to the positive effects of meditation, have hippocampuses on par with regular exercisers. The Dalai Lama himself claims to devote 80 percent of his time to quiet spiritual activities and does not do any organized physical activity. (When Gage chided him about this, the Dalai Lama just let out a big belly laugh.) Later, though, Gage said he and his colleagues found that the monks moved a lot more than they thought, but generally the sort of integrative exercise that all Americans should strive for, such as simply walking to do errands.

Will we ever be able to figure out how to generate healthy neurogenesis in the brain without exercise? Will meditation or even, down the road, a pill, ever do the trick?

The more Dr. Gage pokes around, the more complex the picture becomes and a quick fix for determined sedentary types seems a long way away. Whenever we get our blood circulating at more rigorous levels, for example, we deliver nutrients to the brain that it never receives when we're in a resting state. And something rhythmic begins to happen that mirrors the same brain waves you'd find in the monks while meditating, a synchronization of the mind and body, which researchers are just beginning to unravel.

Indeed, one of the biggest obstacles neuroscientists face is finding ways to measure what they're looking for. How can someone like Dr. Gage know if reading or a run led to the creation of a specific neuron? It took years to fine tune the process that arrived at the answer.

"I believe the organ of maximum impact is our brain," Dr. Gage told me. "And what we do as individuals does change our brains; therefore, we are, in fact, what we do."

And what we were doing for tens of thousands of years was moving; coming to a full stop in our modern adult lives seems akin to throwing ice water on the mind.

14

Reclaiming Natural Grace in Natural Places

Have You Had a Green Hour Today?

I thought God had entered me through the soles of my feet. I was ten and exploring a woodland and trout stream near my new house when I stepped barefoot into the brook. The sensation of snowmelt and pebbles against my skin shook me awake in a way I had never felt before. From that moment on, I couldn't get enough of that place and spent every free moment I had in the water.

My teenage daughter has never experienced this kind of revelation, which only comes if you move through the natural environment on your own and come upon something that startles. The dramatic decline in free-flowing physical activity among children in America has led to an even more astonishing drop in their contact with the natural world. Eighty percent of Americans live in metro areas today, which would seem to explain the trend, but I lived just outside of Hartford, Connecticut, at the time of my woodland meanderings, which put me squarely under the "metro living" category, but I still found my way to willow tree and stream bed.

The more telling statistic is the tremendous reduction in the circle of free movement among kids today. A ten-year-old in 1970 wandered *nine to ten times* as far on his or her own than a ten-year-old today. Saddled by society's often irrational fear of woodlands and many public parks, as well as a huge uptick in indoor recreational options, including video games, cable TV, and instant messaging on the computer, my daughter never makes it to the two streams near our home.

Even if she did find her way there, she wouldn't discover much of interest because pollution has killed off most of the stream life. My brook had crawfish, trout, turtles, frogs, insects that walked on water, dragonflies, footprints in the sand from fox, raccoon, and deer, appalling leeches that occasionally latched onto my ankles, snakes, and hundreds of things that I saw but could give no name.

While biking along a river on a warm June evening, I noticed hardly any insects smacked my shirt and face as I pedaled. All the mosquitoes, gnats, June bugs, and other pesky miniature flyers that swamp creatures love to feed on simply weren't there. I sensed the change because I remember the buggier summers of my youth. My daughter has no such reference point. In truth this pollution-scarred stretch of a river near a city resembles a pristine waterway about as much as a shopping mall resembles a true downtown. The river has its fine points, including splendid views of the distant shoreline and lots of boat traffic, but it lacks organic zest.

To tell the story of how the decline in physical activity has led to a devastating fissure between American children and nature, I decided I needed a cleaner, cooler place to start, a place thick with life, even the stinging variety. So I went to Maine, the state of my maternal ancestors, who worked a rigorous life in the lumber camps there in the late nineteenth and early twentieth centuries.

I stand barefoot in a tidal pool at a place called Popham Beach. It is July, midday, the temperature near eighty degrees, but the North Atlantic waters don't respond quickly to such niceties. The sea beneath me chills my ankles to the winching point. I know from experience that I must wait, that I must allow my body to recognize where I am and what it needs to do to adjust. Miraculously, it always does precisely that, as the pain gives way to numbness, which gives way to feeling and acceptance. I wade deeper; mussels and seaweed with dark green pods cling to the rocks on my right. Popham Beach actually has several small rock "islands"—no bigger than half an acre—which buffet visitors from the open ocean. Standing in my little cove I can hear the surf's aggressive conversation with the granite on the other side. I choose this particular space because, quite frankly, I know I could die around the bend because of the currents, aggressive waves, and intense water temperature. There's a memorial on the ridge to people who drowned because they failed to respect this line.

Children play behind me with a beach ball. The sand bars go on for miles, with pockets of water of varying temperatures in delightful patterns, as though a giant had skipped a stone and left divots here and there.

I admit I am here for my book so I can relive the memory of the extreme cold on the soles of my feet, but I am also here to celebrate the full feeling in my legs. The month following my accident I began to lose sensation and strength in my left leg and no one, not even the surgeon, knew if I could regain it. I press my toes into the sandy bottom, close my eyes, and feel the motion of the tide against my thighs. I experience a sense of vertigo, which I find appealing because it makes me think of the earth rotating on its axis. I am moving way outside of myself into the landscape, which embraces me because I let it. I know I have to be quiet, open, respectful, and patient. I know it will all soothe me—the pungent salty air, the rush of noise pulsating from the waves on the other side, the biting coolness against my skin.

And you, the reader, are probably already restless, wondering when I'll get to the more important information at hand, onto the interviews, facts, government reports, and suggested solutions to the clear crisis that currently exists with regard to American children's lack of direct experience in nature.

But the most important aspect of the story lies here at my feet. I am not talking of the Atlantic, but of the *pace* of my experience. The ocean takes things from me only if I pause and let it. There have been many books and articles about all the practical obstacles that get in the way of children experiencing the outdoors, including an irrational fear of strangers, a lack of wild places, poor access, over-scheduled days, and more. But what good is a child in nature if that child operates at a "civilized" speed, which I use to mean the precise opposite of the original intent of that word? They've developed minds accustomed to a constant stream of stimuli from cell phones, television, iPods playing music in their ears, and computers. At the same time, they deny the needs of their young bodies while they sit to stimulate their minds.

When my daughter's middle school class went on a camping trip, the kids certainly spent time in nature. They camped in tents, ate by a fire, and spent the night near a beach. But they brought their "civilized" mindset to the experience, which meant they wanted to sit, not swim, hike, or explore. They sat on their logs the same way they sit in front of their computers and complained about being bored. The adults in their lives failed to see that simply placing them in nature is not enough; they need to be trained to embrace a natural mindset when they are there, one that respects the pace of tidal pools and seasons. At first it seems impossible because they have so little exposure to nature, but if a kid can follow a baseball game and also appreciate the speed of an ice hockey game, then it's doable.

So precisely how "quick" have their daily lives become? On a physical level, of course, they rarely move at a moderate level for more than an hour a day. But if I measure sound, light, and visual stimulation, they race along at a migraine-inducing rate. The average American household keeps the television on seven hours a day. Children only sit down and actually watch for about three hours a day—a figure that has remained pretty constant over the years— but now they also tag on video games and the computer. The total sit-down time in front of an over-stimulating visual "field" can account for as much as 50 percent or more of the average American child's daily life.

And what of the noise, which I cannot re-create on this flat page? It's not unrealistic to imagine a thirteen-year-old listening to an I-Pod while she talks on her cell phone with the TV on in the background. A whisper registers about thirty decibels; a form of measurement that works on a logarithmic not arithmetic scale so a ten decibel increase means ten times as much sound. According to the Environmental Protection Agency, humans can listen to about seventy decibels on average over a twenty-four-hour period without damaging their hearing, which is a pretty lax standard that doesn't take into account sleep loss, mental stress, and general annoyance. I conjecture that at the precise moment the teen gets on the phone, she creates a situation where she's hearing perhaps as much as ninety decibels (on par with a noisy pub). If she stood quietly in a woodland on a sunny day she'd hear the sound of leaves rustling at about forty-five decibels. When I did the math, those special whistles that only dogs can hear immediately came to mind; only this time the whistle is nature and we can't hear it.

The other arm in the troika of sensory damage comes from the constant use of lights, which illuminate the American landscape so intensely that migrating birds often get disoriented while traveling up and down the East coast because they can't tell what time of day it is or accurately read the landscape on their routes. The same glare shakes us from our natural biorhythms as well, disturbing sleep, moods, and energy levels.

In the end the chronic over-stimulation of the senses and misuse of the physical body leaves the average American child in a weird state of physical torpor, mental overload, and sensory shutdown. No wonder the kids sat on the log at the campsite. They must turn a blind eye and deaf ear, but somehow sustain a revved mind to survive their technology-charged environments. Those same traits leave them almost inert in a natural setting.

Why does it matter? As long as they can navigate the man-made world, perhaps seeing a trout in a stream is irrelevant. But as Richard Louv points out in his book, *Last Child in the Woods,* it's no coincidence that the obesity epidemic mirrored the boom in organized sports. People who have more opportunities to move freely throughout the landscape, especially the natural landscape, have much greater overall health. Children who struggle with everything from depression to attention-deficit disorder generally improve if given the opportunity to move even one hour a day in a green area. In some instances, that one simple "treatment" makes medication unnecessary. One study showed that girls who simply *saw* greenery outside their window overcame their depression quicker.

Humans evolved in nature and remain hardwired right down to the molecular level to exist at a pace that fits in the natural world. When we stop moving through meadows, no longer trek mountain trails or footpaths, we deny not only our physical legacy but our place in the natural world. Louv calls Americans' dependency on over-stimulating televisions and computers a form of "cultural autism," a term that ideally describes the body language and mental state of the seventh graders on the field trip. They might as well have been watching spinning cans.

Louv also points out that children increasingly relate to the natural world in the abstract. They go to the Rain Forest Café for lunch or donate money to save the gorillas in Rwanda, but they never check to see if the hummingbird made it to their backyard feeder this year. If they don't check the feeder, how will they know what's missing, which brings us right back to the insect-free swamp story. Too many Americans have a very sterile vision of what constitutes "normal" in nature, a point of view that will eventually kill our planet if we're not careful. An insect-free world is not a healthy world, no matter how much we may hate the gnats.

In *The Geography of Childhood: Why Children Need Wild Places,* Gary Paul Nabhan talks about how the natural world does not judge and encourages playfulness and spontaneity. "The vocation of being a naturalist on one's home ground is truly the oldest profession in the world." He calculated that during his years of public schooling his teachers brought his class out into "the marvelous natural laboratory" of places like dunes or forests for hands-on learning just a handful of hours each year. For the current school-age generation of Americans, the total is probably even less, especially in urban areas.

"Our world today is one in which we are losing ways of speaking about plants and animals as rapidly as we are losing endangered species themselves," Nabhan concludes. Natural folklore is dying out. There are no new nature stories taking their place, no continuation of the 10,000-year-old narrative that humans have sustained and added to for generations.

Americans built their national sense of self on the backs of mythical characters like the woodsmen Paul Bunyan and Davy Crockett, or the ax-wielding George Washington and Abraham Lincoln. The fact they lived in the wilderness, survived and even thrived, and emerged as leaders of men is a tale told again and again in those same schools that never take students into nature. I vividly remember reading about Paul Bunyan and his blue ox Babe in grade school. The muscular, savvy, good-tempered, fearless, fair woodsman could clear whole forests with a swing of his ax and once leveled twelve acres of jack pine by simply blowing on a whistle.

I so embraced the notion of the physically imposing character moving through nature that I often pretended to be Tarzan, Robin Hood, or even Pippi Longstocking, the Swedish girl with the red braids and superhuman strength, when I played around the stream. I truly believed that being sure-footed, adept in the woods, and an independent roamer in the world were all hallmarks of a superior character. No person of substance would go through life without learning how to be in nature with confidence and style. The history books at school, with their tales of conquering the west, backed me up.

Now even these romanticized visions of Americans in nature have begun to fade. Who needs big forearms or an ax today? My daughter doesn't even know one person who chops wood regularly or works in the outdoors daily. While my own grandfather grew up in a lumbering camp in Maine, lugging water and dodging logs on the Penobscot River, my daughter has no living relative who worked that close to the land. She represents the first generation of Americans with no direct engagement with the outdoors and no living relatives who had a direct engagement with the outdoors.

Again, how much does it matter? In 2005 in an effort to stem criticism that video games encourage kids to be too sedentary, the industry created a new category called "exergaming," which includes the incredibly popular Wii. Players are certainly more physically active than their key-punching counterparts, and they're interacting with others and maybe even with their parents. They work up a sweat and certainly have fun.

But I reaffirmed for myself that things have gotten oddly skewed in the fitness world when I recently had a conversation with a woman who supervises a huge county park and recreation program. While chatting idly, I mentioned that I planned to bike along the river.

"Oh, you like to exercise *outside?*" she asked.

She said the last word as though "outside" were some sort of special niche, which makes sense because most of the activities she directs, like aerobics or spinning classes, take place indoors in gyms, exercise rooms, or pools. But for most of my life when someone said they were going to exercise or play, it implied "outside." I distinctly remember the look in my mother's green eyes when she made it clear that it was time to go "play." She did not mean in the living room.

The link between movement and the outdoors was assumed and inviolate. Now most play and activity takes place in the vacuum of a room with four walls, a trend I call the cauterization of fitness.

I confess, I wish I could have listened to music on something as slick and small as an iPod shuffle when I was a kid. I think it's fantastic that my daughter can reach outside of her small social group at school simply by going to MySpace online and establishing new "virtual" friendships with other girls all over the country who share some of her interests.

But despite such sympathy, even envy, I must bring you back to the cold Atlantic water again. I must turn your eye outward, outside walls, outside the gossip and the latest hot tune. Something much bigger than batteries and electricity drives the experience out here as I watch the late afternoon tide pull away and hope to catch sight of a seal.

If I asked most Americans if they'd be fulfilled and happy if they could shop in malls, work out to videos, and never step outside again, the majority would say "no." We know at a gut level we need some relationship with the natural world or else our growing indifference and ignorance will destroy our planet.

As Louv and others have shown in their books and articles, the number of obstacles keeping children from playing freely outdoors is astounding and growing: public parks that require special use permits to even play catch on an open field; school programs cutting back on recess; hyperventilating parents afraid to let their kids outside alone, who then push them into endless organized activities instead (which means those outside areas really are desolate); a growing number of climate-controlled indoor play areas, etc. No matter how rich the high-tech play world becomes, there's no way to justify demonizing outdoor free play as something that's unsafe and no longer possible in most metro areas for children under age fourteen.

Fortunately hundreds of organizations are fighting back with programs that specifically focus on getting children outdoors more frequently in truly green areas like streams and woodlands not just asphalt playgrounds. Before I went to Maine, I visited the director of one of these programs, Kevin Coyle, who oversees the Green Hour for the National Wildlife Federation, a national conservation organization headquartered in Reston, Virginia.

While I wait for Kevin, I spy the bicycles that NWF puts in the lobby for its employees to use during their lunch breaks. While the headquarters itself is housed in a nondescript building in a nondescript suburban office park, there are excellent bicycle trails nearby and a large woodland in the back, further evidence that people can find ways to be in nature just about anywhere if they just make the effort. Clearly NWF wants its employees to make the effort.

Kevin gives me a firm handshake. A robust middle-aged man with blue eyes and a graying goatee and mustache, he begins by telling me about his firsthand experience with multiple generations in his own household. He currently deals with his kids, his wife's kids and grandchildren, who all fall between the age of ten to thirty-five.

"I can see this huge generational shift. The kids who are under age twenty-one are always online. At dinner they probably get ten cell phone calls. The TV is on in the background; the computer is on; they are text messaging. My granddaughter is almost never outside. She's really physically out of shape and has no stamina.

"So the world these kids live in most of the time is super-velocity, super-agitated. The question I ask myself is how can we get them to this other world, like the banks of the Potomac [River]?"

On a sheet of lined paper, he draws a nickel-sized box to represent the indoors and a second box to represent nature. He runs a vertical line between the two of them. As he moves his hand back and forth over that line, his eyes actually focus on some point in front of him, as though he is trying to envision in his head what it takes to literally get those kids onto the banks of the river.

"My experience is if you can get them past it [he points to the line] and out there [he points to the 'nature' box] they are fine."

When I first heard about the Green Hour program I figured it aimed to get people outside in nature at least sixty minutes a week. But Kevin Coyle and NWF are far more ambitious than that. They know people should get an hour of activity everyday, so they reason, why not combine the physical activity goals with outdoor activities and have a green hour *everyday*?

The website provides advice for parents on how to get kids of any age outside in nature in just about any neighborhood environment. It also runs news flashes and fact sheets that let visitors know things like:

- 60 percent of children ages two to five do not have daily access to outdoor play.
- California started a statewide outdoor education program for schools funded by license plate fees.

◉   Researchers at Cornell University found that kids who play outdoors regularly prior to age eleven are much more apt to grow up to be "environmentally oriented adults"—in other words, good stewards of the earth.

The Green Hour page even offers suggestions on how "Soccer Moms" can become "Fishing Moms."

But after crisscrossing the country for my book, I know firsthand that most Americans do not find an hour in their day to move, never mind outside. Most schoolyards have a dirt field and asphalt playing area, so even if the Green Hour program succeeds in regaining more recess time nationwide (a laudable goal), the kids will not be outside in nature as NWF defines it.

Kevin faces my skepticism with a well-honed stoicism. He's heard it all before, I'm certain, but he presses on. Why can't we have a "No Child Left Inside" type of national program, he asks? I like this twist on President Bush's educational slogan. I like its big attitude and ambition. Perhaps thinking in sweeping, aggressive terms is the only way. Bring back recess *and* overhaul playgrounds so they include green spaces again. Why not link the two agendas, just as I feel we need to link the push for more physical activity with the need to reconnect with nature?

Before I leave, Kevin returns to stories of his own children and grand-children. They will always live in a wired world, he says; that's not going to change, so whatever he does in his program he must work around that. When I ask him about the mindset they need to survive in that wired world and how paralyzing that mindset can be in the quiet of the natural landscape, he nods. I can see that he hasn't thought that much about this second issue: how to give children the skills they need to sit in nature without being bored, restless, or physically inert. Can they truly learn to move through the two universes the way a spectator moves from a baseball game to an ice hockey game?

"You have to have faith that by physically getting the person into the field, into the woods, onto the beach, they will undergo the experience themselves and make the transition themselves," he responds. He admits that one hour a day probably won't do the trick and that most kids need to go into nature for days on end before they "detox" from their overcharged wired-worlds and settle down enough to really embrace the outdoor experience.

I do believe at some point it's too late. As the Cornell study showed, if a parent doesn't instill a connection between a child and the outdoors by the time the child is eleven or so, it appears almost impossible to establish the link. The science writer Rachel Carson addressed this tipping point in her final book, *The Sense of Wonder*, published more than thirty years ago, way before the high-tech wave.

She first became nationally famous for her book, *Silent Spring*, which laid out for the American public in plain English the horrible consequences of flooding our environment and our homes with pesticides, insecticides, and other chemicals. Her work raised such a ruckus the federal government created the Environmental Protection Agency and essentially pulled many of the chemicals, including DDT, off the American market.

In the much lighter *Sense of Wonder*, Carson chronicles the walks she took with her young nephew Roger, whom she helped raise. Instead of reporting on the breakdown of the relationship between nature and man, she lovingly pieces together how to craft a bond between a child and the natural world. The middle-aged Aunt Rachel, who died young at age fifty-six of breast cancer, and the young boy made their way around the coastline of Southport Island in Maine, where Carson spent her summers at a cottage she bought in 1946.

She especially liked going out at night to see ghost crabs, phosphoric scent creatures in the waves, and other nocturnal surprises.

"It was hardly a conventional way to entertain one so young," she admits, "but now, with Roger a little past his fourth birthday, we are continuing that sharing of adventures in the world of nature that we began in his babyhood and I think the results are good. The sharing includes nature in storm as well as calm, by night as well as day, and is based on having fun together rather than on teaching."

Later in the text she acknowledges that most adults feel they have "little nature lore at their disposal" but pushes that aside as a feeble excuse for not getting out there to see the stars, clouds, surf, and changing light. Even in an apartment building, a person can watch the rain.

"Exploring nature with your child is largely a matter of becoming receptive to what lies all around you. It is learning again to use your eyes, ears, nostrils, and finger tips, opening up the disused channels of sensory impression."

In the end, Carson counsels, a person must move through nature at an early age to develop "a sense of wonder so indestructible that it would last throughout life."

And that was precisely what touched me in that cold stream when I was ten; a sense of wonder so profound it felt spiritual.

While in Maine I tried to track down Rachel Carson's small vacation cottage on Southport Island just outside of Boothbay. I wondered if I could walk along the rocky outcrops precisely where this woman had made tidepooling a verb in her life. I did learn that her nephew Roger still owns the place, but it remains private. No one could give me precise directions, though Mainers are famously stingy with local news and may have been protecting the family's privacy. I drove along the heavy-forested side of the island that I thought she probably lived on and went down a small road to the public boat landing. I stood on the dock in the summer sun on a clear day and watched the boats move in and out of the inlet. It was a picture-perfect Maine coastal scene, complete with pine-covered small islands, lots of rock, and cold, clear water. Carson had to be mighty nimble to navigate this unforgiving blend of slippery seaweed and stone.

But she did, often with flashlight in hand, as she returned a starfish at night at low tide or simply lay there with a friend to watch the stars. Whenever she could, she brought Roger with her, never thinking he would be bored or tire. For Carson, being outside was being.

How can I teach that to my own daughter as she instant messages her friends while humming to some tune on her iPod? Every year I take her to a cottage in New Hampshire, though other parents have warned me that once kids reach their teen years they will only enjoy it if they have a friend. Now that she's a teen, I may find that the landscape alone, the time in the rowboat on the lake picking blueberries by herself, will no longer sustain her attention.

But I remain confident that I can find ways to bring her into the land and sea, into the sun and wind, into the night. My greatest fear is that she will lose her capacity to be *in* those places because the modern lifestyle will have pounded her natural senses nearly senseless. The only way a national "No Child Left Inside" program could work is if it included a meditative component that teaches children to shift with the pace of their surroundings.

In her will, Rachel Carson requested that some of her ashes be scattered around her cottage on Southport, and that her family read from T.S. Eliot's "The Four Quartets." I look it up and find to my delight that the strand of lines that they read focused on following nature's time and rhythms, not the slap, dash, and stir of modern life. A tolling bell in the fog, "Measures time not our time, rung by the unhurried / Ground Swell . . . / When time stops and time is never ending."

When I put the soles of my feet in the cold waters of the summer surf of Maine, I enter into that time. I want my daughter and her friends and her children to be able to enter there with me, because it heals, because it revitalizes, because, on some level, it is God under the soles of our feet.

Final Stop

As my own body healed after my bicycle accident, I became more aware of the wounded national body and felt compelled to write *American Idle*. When I could do little more than walk around the block each day after my back surgery, I realized that my physical life had contracted to the same space that most Americans live in. I was stunned that the average person voluntarily gave up so much physical zest and pleasure.

I knew from the start that I did not want to write a book that repeated the same mantra—eat less and exercise more—because that line of attack hasn't budged the 65 percent of Americans who still don't do either. As I traveled around the country, I became convinced that everyone was asking the wrong questions, focusing on the wrong consequences, and talking about the entire problem sideways instead of head on. Issues like body weight and heart rate certainly count for something, but the incredible decline in physical activity in the United States has ripped apart our civic life, further demoralized struggling low-income populations, undermined our collective morality, and has created a devastating rift between human society and nature.

Things started looking grim as soon as the desk-job culture took hold in the nineteenth century. Unfortunately, the instinct to respond to the physical fallout of an industrial society with an equally practical, almost mechanical, approach to fitness, which celebrated measurable things like record times and competitive victories just exacerbated the problem in the long run. By placing physical activity "out there" as something we choose to do for recreation or for competition further distanced us from the fact that movement should be as integral to a person's day as sleep. Most weight loss and fitness programs are fundamentally flawed because they make participants feel as though they are doing a chore or reaching a goal. As Dr. Gage at the Salk Institute showed in his research, exercising under duress actually negates many of the positive effects of the exercise.

Humans physically moved through the landscape for tens of thousands of years and never once thought of measuring their mileage, checking their weight loss or comparing their muscles. And when we placed fitness out there we put nature with it. With each succeeding generation, children spend less time in gardens, around streams, in woodlands, and around any type of creature beside house pets. The rise in organized sports, with its emphasis on structured activities, coincided with the rise in obesity, as people became less and less at home with free play and other spontaneous movement. In the same way, the increased focus on indoor life and entertainment has coincided with global warming and a general destruction of natural habitat. The more out-of-touch we become with our bodies and our place in the natural cycle of life, the more out of balance every aspect of our life becomes, not just our weight or blood pressure.

Study after study shows that adults who physically move throughout their day, right down to fidgeting around the house, live longer lives and have sharper minds. There's a direct correlation between energy expended and life expectancy, with the more active individuals dying at significantly lowers rates than the sedentary types. What's so remarkable about these findings is that a person doesn't have to engage in an organized exercise class or sport to enjoy the benefits; simply vacuuming, taking the stairs, or even walking around the neighborhood works as well.

I know personally whenever I am distressed I always resort to movement, ideally outside in nature, to calm myself. No matter the depth of the tragedy, I can always count on my body to recharge my spirit. I simply hop on my bicycle, walk a few miles, or shoot hoops in silence, anything that gets my skin to sweat, my muscles to contract, and my heart rate to rise. As I showed in Chapter Two, "The History of the Body as Told by the Body," if you don't move but eat a lot your body thinks you're gorging in a time of famine and holds pounds and withdraws physically and emotionally. Physical activity of any kind tells the most primitive part of your brain that you are needed, engaged, and well.

On a daily basis more than 60 percent of Americans fail to send this message to themselves, a lifestyle travesty of astounding proportions that will require a radical fix that involves not just individuals accepting personal responsibility, but also schools, employers, and urban planners. As Dr. Ornish's study made clear, aggressive changes done within the context of a supportive group produce the most lasting results.

So what should those changes be and how do Americans create support groups on a local scale?

The first part of that question remains the most contentious. I heard a cacophony of health advice while on my road trip, from the National Institutes of Health (NIH) announcements on the radio to the advertisements for ab machines on my TV at home. Most of it made physical activity sound like something people engage in only during inspired moments.

Americans need to reclaim movement as a natural part of their daily lives, an approach to fitness often called Integrative Exercise.

The focus needs to shift away from organized classes and sports and toward sustaining an active flow of movement throughout the day. With this criteria as the baseline, then the walkability of a town or the chance for light movement breaks at work takes on just as much importance as whether or not a person has access to an aerobics class three times a week.

Sharon Roerty of the National Center for Bicycling & Walking made it clear that this "flow" I seek begins on the streets of American towns, many of which need to be redesigned to encourage people to move on their own two feet again. At least the federal government put some money and muscle behind the idea of getting more children to walk to their local public schools, though $612 million for the Safe Routes to Schools program should be seen as a start not an end unto itself. A recent study showed that kids who engage in light exercise before exams, like a one-mile walk, performed 25 percent better than their counterparts who were tutored for the same amount of time. Perhaps declining standardized test scores in American schools have as much to do with blood flow as with overworked, undersupplied teachers.

Hundreds of organizations in the public and private sector have taken up walkable landscapes as a cause celebre with great success and most new developments in major metro areas now worry about being pedestrian-friendly. But these changes, and many others necessary to make it easier for Americans to move more freely on a physical level on a daily basis, remain voluntary.

At a health assembly in 2004, the World Health Organization (WHO) issued a report titled, "Strategy for Diet, Physical Activity and Health," which addressed the global drop in physical activity among humans, especially in affluent cultures, and *projected that 73 percent of global deaths worldwide would result from poor lifestyle choices by the year 2020.* Their answer: get governments on board and make *gradual* changes in diet and physical-activity patterns. They listed goals, such as thirty minutes of moderate activity every day, and suggested ways for governments and public-health officials to get started.

This soft shoe approach clearly didn't work. When WHO did a follow up study to assess the success of the 2004 plan, it found evidence of little progress. The 2006 report dropped the word *gradual* and replaced it with "more needs to be done—*urgently.*" (Emphasis added.)

Other well-intentioned organizations have bumped up against the same problems after they issue their intelligent, on-target suggestions and then wait for something to happen. The same year that WHO issued its global plan, the Institute of Medicine in the United States came out with a scathing report about obesity and claimed it had reached epidemic levels and that radical changes had to take place at every level of society. "I think we need to make a revolution," said Dr. Jeffrey Kaplan, chair of the commission behind the report, which emphasized the need for more physical education in schools, stricter guidelines for marketing food to children, etc. But every suggestion was couched with "should" or "could" rather than "must."

Voluntary won't work. The reports and suggestions from the Institute of Medicine and WHO, and countless other organizations desperately trying to get Americans and even the global population to listen, have had a modest impact. They certainly provide a workable outline, but the real deal will only

happen when there's the political will at every level—local, state, and federal—
and a call for personal responsibility.

Going back to Dr. Ornish's claim that radical change is the only way
to go, think of how we eradicated smoking from most public transportation.
People simply don't light up in busses, trains, and airplanes anymore, even
though a good 20 percent of Americans want to. The sheer volume of local,
state, and federal laws, and the sheer volume of stories that made it clear that
even second-hand smoke is deadly brought about a societal shift of astounding
scale and effectiveness.

The word on how to improve our lifestyle habits is already out there;
the will is not. We need to use the law to make the changes that we have such
trouble making on an individual level. The laws don't have to be draconian,
just firm. Sharon Roerty gave a fine example when she pointed out that every
major town resurfaces its roads on a ten-year cycle. Why not *require* towns
to incorporate bicycle lanes and pedestrian-friendly changes on every major
thoroughfare as part of their resurfacing plan? They have to do the job either
way and redrawing the lines for the space won't really cost more money. It's a
matter of priorities, not cash.

The Utz Potato Chip factory managers realized, when possible, they
needed to move their workers to new stations every thirty minutes to balance
out the employees' overall body movements throughout the day. Why can't
industries such as law, insurance, and other desk-dependent work places take a
similar approach and allocate two fifteen-minute *movement* breaks within each
eight-hour work cycle?

On the face of it, these suggestions seems pretty innocuous, but Americans are notorious for balking at anything that smacks of control when it
comes to their lifestyle choices. While I haven't spoken much about diet in this
book, the eating/exercise axis lies at the center of Americans' collective health
issues. The more I looked at our physical-activity patterns, the more I kept
bumping up against fat, both in our diet and on our bodies. Too many calories
+ not enough exercise = an overweight populace is a pretty basic equation and
certainly a very fixable one.

But we can't even muster the communal will to get unhealthy snack food
out of public school vending machines. Educators, parents, and politicians

know that school lunches in most places, with their canned fruit in corn syrup and pizza specials, are a national embarrassment that run completely counter to all the talk about making healthier lifestyle choices. I admit, with some relief, that political will *is* building: In 2005 alone, legislators considered more than 200 bills in forty states that sought to ban soda and junk food from schools. In 2007 Dr. Farley and the CDC launched their ambitious PACE program in New Orleans.

But for real change to take effect, Americans need to embrace a new axis made up of *political will and personal responsibility*.

The federally subsidized lunch program currently allocates just $3.50 per student per day for breakfast *and* lunch. The schools in Rome, Italy, shell out $5 per kid a day for lunch and 70 percent of the ingredients the children eat are organic.

Put another way, as Burkhard Bilger pointed out in his *New Yorker* article, "The Lunchroom Rebellion," the U.S. government subsidy for school lunches runs about $7 billion a year. The war in Iraq runs us more than a billion dollars a week.

Political will and personal responsibility.

When renowned chef Ann Cooper agreed to step out of the rarefied world of fine cuisine to become the top lunch lady in Berkeley's public school system in California, she hoped to revolutionize what kind of food American kids could eat on a mass scale. But as Bilger shows in his article, Cooper struggled as she battled entrenched attitudes among old staffers and—well for lack of a better word—damaged palates in American kids.

Cooper teamed with a top baker to create a whole wheat, organic, vegetarian pizza, but the students didn't like it and demanded the return of the more traditional variety. Parents and many school administrators sided with the students and the Cooper pizza was pulled.

Political will and personal responsibility.

Oddly enough, much of the world is making the same choice as the Berkeley crowd and opting for American fast food and physical-activity patterns, even though it's obvious that our way is not the healthier way.

Sweden offers an excellent prototype of what can work, what we all struggle to sustain, and the forces that keep pressuring us in the wrong direction.

On the enviable side of the equation, Swedish children ages six to twelve do 20 percent more physical activity than their American counterparts. They have more recess and less class time but beat us on standardized tests in math and English. In the workplace, nearly 20 percent of Swedish employees are allowed to take exercise breaks as part of their *paid working hours.*

But instead of the U.S. emulating Sweden, the Swedes are emulating us and increasing their intake of fast food and slowly dropping their physical-activity levels. The result: the percentage of overweight Swedish kids has risen to 18 percent (compared to 32 percent in the U.S.) and the number of hours the average adult works each week continues to increase as the country struggles to stay competitive in global markets.

Studies show that *required, paid movement breaks* at work have the highest success rate as measured by steady participation and overall improved health and work performance. The U.S. model of not offering anything or pushing for wellness-related activities before and after work or during the unpaid lunch break simply don't measure up. And yet Sweden and the rest of the globe have had an alarming tendency to follow the American lead, a trend that helped contribute to WHO's dire predictions about lifestyle-related health problems on a global scale.

Again, the infrastructure for effective change exists right under our noses. The U.S. Department of Labor's web page has a section about "Break and Meal Periods," which explains that federal law does not require coffee breaks, but when an employer does offer short breaks (usually five to twenty minutes) "federal law considers *the break work time that must be paid.*" Just replace the word "coffee" with "movement" and Americans would have the makings of a federally sanctioned *paid* exercise break.

As things stand now, under "Breaks" the USDL lists things like Flexible Schedules, Holidays, and Job Sharing, but nothing about wellness or fitness. Physical activity is simply not even included under the province of that word.

There is one government agency that Americans can turn to for a prototype on how to alter lifestyle patterns on a society-wide scale and get the masses into reasonable shape again: the military. For centuries, in cultures around the world, leaders have sweated over how to keep their young men in fit, fighting order. Bill Sands from the U.S. Olympic Center reminded me that gymnastics evolved in Europe in the early nineteenth century because the German military wanted a way to keep its soldiers in shape even while on a campaign. They invented the pommel horse (very portable) and created exercise routines that centered on mats and bars.

In the 1950s, when the United States began to fret about the declining health of its youth, President Eisenhower created the President's Council on Youth Fitness (now called the President's Council for Physical Fitness and Sport) and had a conference at the U.S. Naval Academy. When members of the council wanted to develop a concrete plan of action, they turned to West Point.

Even today, unfit or overweight soldiers are denied access to the professional development schools vital to their progress through the ranks. Granted, I'm talking about healthy young men and women in the prime of their life. It would be impossible to expect every reasonably healthy American under age fifty-five to run two miles in 15 minutes or less and crank out fifty-nine sit-ups in two minutes (Army standards). But the *collective expectation* that every soldier must sustain a certain level of physical activity and overall fitness is worth emulating.

Why can't we set standards for ourselves as a nation, especially in terms of the amount of time we engage in moderate physical movement on a daily basis? Why can't we set a national goal of sixty minutes of movement every day for every adult and child and work to create school environments, work environments, and landscapes that nurture this *collective expectation*?

Political will and personal responsibility.

Our lifestyle choices say volumes about what we value as a culture. Before Integrative Exercise can move to the forefront of the move movement, Americans must learn to care more about a different set of numbers. Right now most people measure their fitness by looking at their weight and body-fat levels, very egocentric and individual concerns. But under the Integrative Exercise umbrella, a person would also care about the amount of time their kids had for free play outdoors, the amount of time they themselves had in the sun, and the chances for simple movement breaks at work that enhance concentration, lower blood pressure, and improve mood. These numbers should matter to Americans as much as their cholesterol readings.

At the Active Living Research Conference in San Diego, the conference attendees didn't burn a lot of calories when they stood up to do Toni Yancey's "Liftoff L.A. Style" routine after breakfast, but the activity did lighten the mood in the room, made everyone more social, and provided wonderful relief to my back after hours in a ninety-degree position on an airplane and in a chair.

Which brings me to my next declaration.

Americans need to assert their right to joyful, recuperative movement.

As Karen Bradley of the Laban/Bartenieff Institute of Movement pointed out in my chapter on the moral consequences of a sedentary life, most people turn to some form of media when they want to relax and recover from their day, but that's probably not the best choice, especially for children. We allow so much visual and audio stimulation in our life that we crowd out any chance to discover a way to decompress that makes sense to us personally.

Before television, our ancestors used their hands constantly during their leisure hours to carve wood, sew, garden, can food, paint, or tinker in general. The poet and novelist D.H. Lawrence captured the beauty of such homespun creations in his poem "Things Men Have Made," in which he describes "things men have made with wakened hands, and put soft life into, are awake through years with transferred touch." I can't imagine him writing that about anything that you could craft or do at a computer.

And we need to breathe "soft life" out of ourselves, which is a form of creative energy that manifests itself in art, dance, even sports, but rarely in daily activities in American life. Part of the problem remains the terrific pace that we all sustain every day, especially mentally. Creativity requires quiet and space, and Americans need to care more about carving that out for themselves at work, at home, and at school for their children. Every public school curriculum should require a meditative moment in the daily schedule, be it outside as part of a green hour, or inside as part of a more prayer-like experience. Until Americans *face* the *pace* problem, the shift to a more integrative approach to exercise will be difficult to accomplish.

As Bradley noted, we're losing our rhythm as a culture. Our sense of time and space has become completely skewed by media and a lack of overall body awareness. Each of us needs to step back out of the noise and piece together a portrait of our ideal physically graceful self. This grace not only encompasses the sort of fine lines we see in a ballet dancer, but also how physical-activity patterns impact social life, moral sensibility, empathy for the natural world, and spirituality.

I know the journey I took to write this book made me step back and reassess every aspect of my personality and body. I am a different person now, here, on this page, than I was when I typed the first paragraph of my Introduction.

I began with the mindset of a frustrated injured athlete, of a thin, white woman who could never figure out why so many Americans put on so much weight and cared so little about their physical health. I began this book thinking I had excellent ideas on how society could heal itself. I smugly assumed I already knew the physical, social, and moral consequences of a sedentary life. I just needed to bear witness.

Instead I end here, my last stop on my journey, humbled by how much physical activity people try to do despite nearly insurmountable obstacles, including unsafe neighborhoods, long work hours, and fast-paced lifestyles. What I learned on my trip upended every assumption I brought to bear on my topic.

I started out thinking that people really needed to do three to five hours of vigorous exercise a week. Now I realize that light amounts of moderate exercise throughout your day every day is a more wholesome approach. You reap the health benefits, are less apt to get injured, and are more apt to stick with it because it's not so goal oriented.

At the start of my project, I still defined my exercise time as a space in my day when I proved myself. Could I make twelve miles on my bike in under an hour? Could I sustain my weight, despite my back surgery and no more basketball? Now, I value a quiet walk that allows me to observe things as particular as insects on a flower. I don't check the time anymore. I just think about the dynamic between my muscles, bones, lungs, and heart and the physical energy I bring to each day. My exercise has become about vitality, not fitness.

I used to have a lively social life at certain basketball courts near where I live. I'd show up for the lunchtime game and played hoops with a sixty-year-old Korean man who once played for the Korean Olympic team, two self-employed white guys who did something on computers, cops from the local county, and a handful of African American men taking a lunch break from their jobs. After hurting my back, I could no longer play and lost contact with all of these people, who were nothing like me. Just after my surgery, I didn't know how I could live without that wonderful rush that comes from pushing your body to its full limits, from executing a pass, a shot, or defensive move that is pure response and artistry.

I never did find something that my back could handle to replace that special rush, but the far greater loss was my *social* contact with the wider world that came to play with me every time I showed up at the courts. While walking the streets of New York City with Sharon Roerty, I faced for the first time how important physical movement can be to our social contacts in society. When we close down public spaces—in my case a public basketball court—we become more insular. Americans remove themselves from their proverbial basketball courts when they stop doing physical activity outside in public areas.

Even at the start of my journey, I knew that children weren't getting outside in nature enough, but I had no concept of the horrible scope of the problem. From the time my daughter could walk, I emphasized outdoor play over indoor play by limiting television and computer time to a bare minimum (almost nonexistent for the first four years). I brought her on camping trips and on hikes up mountains in New England and Colorado. I made sure to dip her feet in the shocking waters of glacier melt. Every summer we spend at least two to three weeks at a cottage on a lake in New Hampshire, where simply making a cup of cocoa involves lugging water (eight pounds a gallon) from a spring, boiling it, drinking the cocoa (bought in a town about thirty minutes away), and finally washing the mugs in lake water then in boiled water. We live deliberately, as Henry David Thoreau might have said, with no TV, computers, one old-fashioned phone (no answering machine), and a good view of the lake and the loons that often wake us with their mournful cries each morning.

But despite my best efforts, despite her genuine affection for outdoor life (she's a terrific kayaker, canoeist, and picker of wild blueberries), it's become increasingly difficult to find things to do with her in nature because, as a teen, she understandably wants company other than her mother, but none of her peers are interested. How can a quiet so profound that we can hear the hummingbird's thrumming wings as he pulls up to our feeder compete with the Wii or even an iPod? It can only compete if a child has already embraced and felt the sense of wonder that Rachel Carson spoke of. Unfortunately, not enough parents put enough value on that particular aspect of their child's education.

I am confident that my daughter will care for nature and be protective of the natural landscape and all of the various creatures in it all of her adult life; but from a social perspective, I'm not sure who will want to share the outdoor spaces with her, and I fear the power of that loneliness. When I think back to the middle school campout, where she surfed the waves and explored a few of the trails, I realize she did almost all of that on her own, while the others sat back at camp.

As I pushed through the final chapters of my book and began looking at the spiritual and moral consequences of a sedentary life, I underwent a change of opinion so complete that I had trouble writing the chapters. I'd start in one place, such as assuming that low-income African Americans and Hispanics just need to make better choices, and wind up wrestling myself into another place altogether. The very groups that I found most baffling when I started, I found most impressive when I finished.

The fact the Hispanics at St. Anthony's Catholic Church, in Arlington, Virginia, make any time whatsoever for a healthy walk just boggles my mind now that I see how many obstacles they face in their daily lives. The fact many of them do try and do listen just proves to me how deep the need for physical movement really can be.

Without better urban planning (especially more pedestrian-and-bicycle-friendly streets), more safe places (churches are a good start), and community resources, these most at-risk groups will continue to be denied their physical activity rights in America. And that's what it is—a right, directly connected to health and happiness. Personal responsibility does play a part, and they certainly need to do a better job making healthier decisions about their diets in particular, but even in this area, as Dr. Farley pointed out in his talk on New Orleans, access and cost play a huge role—two things people have little control over.

And while I knew I wanted to explore the moral consequences of a sedentary life, I didn't expect to find much there, except perhaps a person's obligation to remain healthy for the larger benefit of society because heavy and inactive people drive up healthcare costs. I never expected to learn that on a *biological* level our mentally over-stimulating modern lives impair our moral judgments or that our sluggish lifestyle decreases neurogenesis in our adult brains.

When I started out, I thought I was tapping into a vein, but instead found myself reaching into a life-sustaining artery clogged by poor city planning, poor access, poor funding, insufficient education, and, most importantly, insufficient urgency. My own book has scared me into a different lifestyle.

Even in my conclusion, I headed in a direction I thought I'd never take. Originally I was going to organize this chapter around Sir Isaac Newton's laws of motion: an object at rest stays at rest; an object that moves along untouched by any other force will continue to move along; and for every action there is an equal and opposite reaction. The breakthroughs made by this seventeenth-century British scientist laid the groundwork for many of the technological advances that shape modern society today, so it seemed only fitting to look at the laws and how they apply to Americans' physical-activity patterns.

But it is precisely this sort of technical approach that has created a distance between ourselves and our bodies and moved physical activity somewhere outside of daily life. I decided I needed an American icon who celebrated our physicality as *integral* to our humanity.

So I turned to Walt Whitman, the nineteenth-century American poet, who worked variously as a carpenter, "wound dresser" in the Civil War, and government employee. He crafted with his hands, experienced a desk job, and saw healthy men's bodies torn apart by disease and gunshot, which, in my opinion, made him an expert judge of the American physical experience.

In "The Body Electric," he wrote:

> But the expression of a well-made man appears not only in his face,
> It is in his limbs and joints also, it is curiously in the joints of his hips and wrists,
> It is in his walk, his carriage of his neck, the flex of his waist and knee, dress does not hide him,
> The strong sweet quality he has strikes through the cotton and broadcloth,
> To see him pass conveys as much as the best poem, perhaps more.

At last, a little sex in a book about the physical American. Though of course Whitman meant so much more than that. He would have celebrated the spirit that drives the optimists and explorers I met along the road, especially Sharon Roerty and her efforts to bring more walking and biking trails to even the most difficult urban areas, and Kevin Coyle, who insists on pressing for a Green Hour every day, because that's precisely what Americans do need even if they don't want to hear it. The poet would applaud the archeologists digging in the dirt of Kansas to find out more about the movement patterns of our ancestors, precisely because the past of those hunter-gatherers is our legacy. As Whitman famously sang in "Song of Myself," we each "contain multitudes" and to tune out the song they left us, in this case within the very muscle and bone structure of our bodies, is to undermine our very being.

In the early stanzas of "Song of Myself," Whitman celebrates "The feeling of health, the full-noon trill, the song of me rising from bed and meeting the sun."

That's what I want for all Americans, the full-noon trill that can only emerge from a healthy body.

The first day I stood at my standup desk and broke free of the chair culture that sets off spasms in my back, I realized I could create new movement patterns without straying too far from what already existed in my daily life. This one simple observation launched the journey around the United States that created *American Idle*.

My bicycle accident took away my life as a competitive athlete, but it gave me a much more balanced physical self that's more concerned with meeting the sun, both outside in nature and within me. That full-noon trill I feel within myself is not just health; it's joy, and that is where the move movement can bring all of us if we let it.

Endnotes

Introduction: Reclaiming Our Physical Selves

(65 percent of Americans overweight or obese) U.S. Department of Agriculture, USDA.gov; U.S. Food and Drug Administration, FDA.gov; Centers for Disease Control and Prevention, CDC.gov

(Current generation lower life expectancy) CDC, National Institute for Aging, and "Death Rate from Obesity Gains Fast on Smoking," *New York Times*, March 10, 2004.

(Life expectancy for hunter-gatherers and lifestyle) Robert Kelly, *The Foraging Spectrum: Diversity in Hunter-Gatherer Lifestyles*, Smithsonian Institute Press, 1995, p. 20; Dr. Chris Ruff, Physiology Department, Johns Hopkins University; on-location interviews in Kanorado, CO, with Dr. Steve Holen, curator, Denver Museum of Nature and Science, and Dr. Rolfe Mandel, professor of geoarcheology, University of Kansas, June 6, 2005.

(Information on the body) Leslie Aiello, et. al., *An Introduction to Human Evolutionary Anatomy*, Academic Press, 1990; John Langdon, *The Human Strategy: An Evolutionary Perspective on Human Anatomy*, Oxford University Press, 2005; "Fatter Than Other Animals," *Economist*, December 13, 2003, p. 5; Chris Crowley and Henry Lodge, *Younger Next Year: A Guide to Living Like 50 Until You're 80 and Beyond*, Workman Publishing, 2004.

(Zoo information and animal-movement patterns) Visit to National Zoo in Washington, DC, and interview with John Gibbons, public affairs, January 4, 2005.

(Sleep averages) Carl Zimmer, "Down for the Count," *New York Times*, November 8, 2005, p. D 1.

(Bear information) Bernd Heinrich, *Winter World: The Ingenuity of Animal Survival*, Ecco, a division of HarperCollins, 2003.

(50 percent of Americans on farms until 1920s) Maury Klein, *The Genesis of Industrial America 1870-1920*, Cambridge Essential History Series, Cambridge University Press, 2007.

(Beecher information) Catherine Beecher, *Letters to the People on Health and Happiness*, Arno Press (originally published 1855).

(History of fitness equipment and college-sports information) Kathryn Grover, *Fitness in American Culture: Images of Health, Sport and the Body*, University of Massachusetts Press, 1989; and Carolyn Thomas de la Pena, *The Body Electric: How Strange Machines Built the Modern American*, New York University Press, 2003.

(Hartford and bicycles) Stephen Goddard, *Colonel Albert Pope and His American Dream Machines: The Life and Times of a Bicycle Tycoon Turned Automotive Pioneer*, McFarland and Co. Publishers, 2000.

(Taylor information and Ford Company) Robert Kanigel, *The One Best Way: Frederick Winslow Taylor*, Viking, 1997.

(Assembly-line tours) On-location tours of assembly lines at Utz Potato Chip factory in Hanover, PA, and Harley-Davidson Factory in York, PA, November 10, 2005.

(Olympic Center and Bill Sands) Interview on location at the USOC, in Colorado, with Bill Sands, director of Sports Science at USOC (June 3, 2005).

(Eisenhower Years) U.S. Department of Agriculture, USDA.gov; Health and Human Services, HHS.gov; Centers for Disease Control and Prevention, CDC.gov

(Quiz results) Centers for Disease Control and Prevention, CDC.gov.nccdphp/dnpa/physical/life/overcome.html

(DC woman) Rachel Winch, in-person interview, Cleveland Park, Washington, DC, March 16, 2008.

(25 percent increase in activity with access) Agency for Healthcare Research and Quality, AHRQ.gov.ppip/activity.html and the Active Living Research Conference materials.

(85 percent better life expectancy from preventive measures; LA 49th in mortality rate) Dr. Thomas Farley, Tulane University and keynote speaker at the February 17, 2006 annual Active Living Research Conference in San Diego, CA, as well as his book, *Prescription for a Healthy Nation: A New Approach to Improving Our Lives by Fixing Our Everyday World*, Beacon Press, 2005. PACE website: SPH.tulane.edu/PRC/pages/CoreResearch/html

(Walking tour of NYC) Sharon Roerty, Executive Director of the National Center for Bicycling & Walking; BikeWalk.org

Jane Jacobs, *The Death and Life of Great American Cities*, The Modern Library, 1993 (original edition, 1961).

(Fitness Ministries) St. Anthony of Padua Catholic Church, Arlington, VA, contact: Georgina Redmond, church nurse, (Hispanic congregation); Mount Olive Church, Arlington, VA, contact: LaVaeda Coulter, Fitness Ministry Director; INOVA Congregational Health Partnership, Peggy Steen.

(80 percent of healthcare costs) Alan Deutschman, "Why is it so darn hard to change our ways?" *Fast Company*, May 2005, pp. 53-62; and Dr. Thomas Farley, *Prescription for a Healthy Nation: A New Approach to Improving Our Lives by Fixing Our Everyday World*, Beacon Press, 2005.

(Brain chemistry/morality) Antonio Damasio, *Descartes' Error: Emotion, Reason and the Human Brain,* Putnam Books, 1994; and interview, Steven Johnson, "Antonio Damasio's Theory of Thinking Faster and Faster: Are the brain's emotional circuits hardwired for speed?" *Discovery*, May 2004.

(Laban/Bartenieff Institute Material) Interview with Karen Bradley. Laban/Bartenieff Institute of Movement, 520 Eighth Ave., Room 304, NY, NY 10018; infor@limsonline.org

(Circle of movement among children) Richard Louv, *Last Child in the Woods: Saving Our Children from Nature-Deficit Disorder,* Algonquin Books of Chapel Hill,

2005, p. 116. He cited a study done by Sanfor Gaster, "Urban Children's Access to Their Neighborhood: Changes Over Three Generations," *Environment and Behavior,* January 1991, pp. 70-85.

Dr. Fred Gage, Salk Institute, La Jolla, California, Personal Interview, June 18, 2008.

Amish standup desk: Standupdesks.com

Chapter One: Meet the First Walkers: *The American Heartland 14,000 Years Ago*

On-location interviews in Kanorado, CO, June 6, 2005, with Steve Holen, curator, Denver Museum of Nature and Science, and Rolfe Mandel, professor of geoarcheology, University of Kansas.

(Theories on how first people arrived) DVD, Scientific American, *Frontiers*, "Coming to America" with Alan Alda, July 2004.

(Average hunter-gatherer life) Robert Kelly, *The Foraging Spectrum: Diversity in Hunter-Gatherer Lifeways,* Smithsonian Institute Press, 1995, p. 20.

(Stone Age energy expenditure) John Ratey and Eric Hagerman, *Spark: The Revolutionary New Science of Exercise and the Brain,* Little, Brown and Company, 2008.

(Atlatls) Tim Cahill, *Hold the Enlightenment,* Vintage Books, 2002, pp. 179-186. Atlatls-n-More.com/TyogaAtlatlAssoc

(Farmer family size) Steve Olson, *Mapping Human History: Discovering the Past Through Our Genes,* 2002.

"Coming to America," DVD.

Robert Kelly, *The Foraging Spectrum: Diversity in Hunter-Gatherer Lifeways,* Smithsonian Institute Press, 1995, p 20.

(Farming vs. hunter-gatherer lifestyle) Jane Peterson, *Sexual Revolutions: Gender and Labor at the Dawn of Agriculture,* Altamira Press, 2002, pp. 4-8.

(Studying changes in physique in humans when switched from hunter-gathering to farming) Dr. Chris Ruff, Physiology Department, Johns Hopkins University.

(Hours farmers worked) David Bassett, "Physical Activity in Old Order Amish," *Medicine and Science in Sports and Exercise,* January 2004.

Chapter Two: What Do Our Bodies Want (and Why)? *The History of the Body as Told by the Body*

(Foot information) Jonathan Shaw, "The Deadliest Sin," *Harvard Magazine,* March-April, 2004, p. 38.

(Three million years as only walkers) Dennis Bramble and Daniel Lieberman, "Endurance Running and the Evolution of Homo," *Nature,* Vol. 432, November 18, 2004, pp. 345-352.

(Fibula/tibia information) Leslie Aiello, et. al, *An Introduction to Human Evolutionary Anatomy,* Academic Press, 1990, p. 405.

(Rib cage and breathing) John Langdon, *The Human Strategy: An Evolutionary Perspective on Human Anatomy,* Oxford University Press, 2005, pp. 212-214.

(Outperform animals in running) Dennis Bramble and Daniel Lieberman, "Endurance Running and the Evolution of Homo," *Nature,* Vol. 432, November 18, 2004, pp. 345-352.

(Differences between sexes) Jeffrey Meldrum and Charles Hilton, editors, *From Biped to Strider: The Emergence of Modern Human Walking, Running and Resource Transport,* Kluwer Academic/Plenum Publisher, 2004.

(Dissipating heat) John Langdon, *The Human Strategy: An Evolutionary Perspective on Human Anatomy*, Oxford University Press, 2005, p. 126 and p. 174.

(Tribes running long distances) Bernd Heinrich, *Why We Run: A Natural History*, Harper/Collins, 2001, p. 174.

(Material on bears and sweat glands) Heinrich, *Why We Run*, p. 174.

(Fat cells information) "Fatter Than Other Animals," *Economist*, December 13, 2003, p. 5.

(Why sedentary in wild) Chris Crowley and Henry Lodge, *Younger Next Year: A Guide to Living Like 50 Until You're 80 and Beyond*, Workman Publishing, 2004, p. 39.

(How body interprets TV watching) Crowley and Lodge, *Younger Next Year*, p. 39; John Langdon, *The Human Strategy: An Evolutionary Perspective on Human Anatomy*, Oxford University Press, 2005; Jonathan Shaw, "The Deadliest Sin," *Harvard Magazine*, March-April, 2004, p. 38.

(Exercise as determinant for long life) Jerry Adler and Anne Underwood, "Starve Your Way to Health," *Newsweek*, January 19, 2004, pp. 51-54; also Chris Crowley and Henry Lodge, *Younger Next Year*, Workman Publishing, 2004, p. 74.

(Human traits in other animals) John Langdon, *The Human Strategy: An Evolutionary Perspective on Human Anatomy*, Oxford University Press, 2005, p. 18 and p. 183.

(Mitochondria) Steve Olson, *Mapping Human History: Discovering the Past Through Our Genes*, Houghton Mifflin, 2002, p. 27; also Chris Crowley and Henry Lodge, *Younger Next Year*, Workman Publishing, 2004, p. 98.

Chapter Three: Physical Grace: *The Olympic Center*

On-location interview at the United States Olympic Center in Colorado Springs, CO, June 3, 2005, with Bill Sands, bioengineer and director of the Sports Sciences Department.

(Rate of improvement in records) *British Medical Bulletin*, "updates on improvement of human athletic performance," Lippi, G., Banfi, G., et. al., July, 2008.

American Health Foundation website: AHF.org

National Center for Chronic Disease Prevention and Health Promotion website: CDC.gov/nccdphp/

(Youngest generation today has lower life expectancy than parents because of lifestyle habits) National Institute of Aging: NIA.nih.gov/

(Only 3 percent of adults exercise through team sport) John Ratey and Eric Spark, *The Revolutionary New Science of Exercise and the Brain*, Little, Brown and Company, 2008, p. 17.

(Kansas information) American Health Foundation website: AHF.org; National Center for Chronic Disease Prevention and Health Promotion website: CDC.gov/nccdphp/

Chapter Four: Flashback: *How Did Work Become Sedentary and Physical Activity Become Leisure?*

(Beecher information) Catherine Beecher, *Letters to the People on Health and Happiness*, Arno Press and the *New York Times* reprint 1972, Charles Rosenberg, editor; *Those Beecher Women: A Look Into the Lives of the Influential 19th Century Sisters*, the *Hartford Courant*, special handout at the Harriet Beecher Stowe House.

(Harriet quotations about Cate) *Those Beecher Women*, p. 22 and p. 3.

(Quotations) Beecher, *Letters to the People on Health and Happiness*, p. 125 and p. 244; and Mary Kelley Boydston and Anne Margolis, editors, *The Limits of Sisterhood: The Beecher Sisters on Women's Rights and Woman's Sphere*, University of North Carolina Press, 1988.

(Cate's summary of health information) Beecher, *Letters to the People on Health and Happiness*, p. 115.

(Boxing, horse racing, etc.) John Hoberman, *Mortal Engines: The Science of Performance and the Dehumanization of Sport*, Free Press, 1992 p. 89.

(Marathon news) Lori Riley, "Kemboi Pours it On," *Hartford Courant*, October 9, 2005, p. A1.

On-location visit to the Harriet Beecher Stowe House, October 8, 2005; materials on the wall, including biographies and map.

(Bicycle history) Stephen Goddard, *Colonel Albert Pope and His American Dream Machines: The Life and Times of a Bicycle Tycoon Turned Automotive Pioneer*, McFarland & Co., Publishers, 2000.

(Stowe hearing noise from factory) Goddard, *Colonel Albert Pope and His American Dream Machines*, p. 93.

(CT Bicycle Club) Connecticut Historical Society, Hartford, CT, Bicycle Club Handbook, 1879 (archives).

(Nickel alloy) Stephen Goddard, *Colonel Albert Pope and His American Dream Machines*, p. 78.

(Ads and number of women riders) Visit to Connecticut Historical Society, October 8, 2005 (archives); Goddard, *Colonel Albert Pope and His American Dream Machines*, p. 96.

(Taylor history) International Bicycle Fund (IBF.com) historic time-line and Goddard, *Colonel Albert Pope and His American Dream Machines*, p. 83.

Mark Twain, "Taming the Bicycle," published in *Mark Twain: Collected Tales, Sketches, Speeches and Essays 1852-1890*, Library of America, 1992.

(Holmes quotation) Carolyn Thomas de la Pena, *The Body Electric: How Strange Machines Built the Modern American*, New York University Press, 2003, p. 27.

(Pulling bows) Thomas de la Pena, *The Body Electric*, p. 23, and Hugh Cunningham, *Leisure in the Industrial Revolution*, St. Martin's Press, 1980, p. 60.

(Dr. Sargent) Kathryn Grover, *Fitness in American Culture: Images of Health, Sport and the Body 1830-1940*, University of Massachusetts Press and the Strong Museum in Rochester, NY, 1989, p. 146-47 (information about college campuses), p. 143.

(Physical education as hygiene) John Hoberman, *Mortal Engines: The Science of Performance and the Dehumanization of Sport*, Free Press, 1992, p. 88.

(Dr. Sargent) Carolyn Thomas de la Pena, *The Body Electric: How Strange Machines Built the Modern American*, New York University Press, 2003, pp. 56-57; and Boston University website, historical section.

(Author's mother) Connie Sullivan Collins Cain, Farmington, CT.

(Pope Park) Stephen Goddard, *Colonel Albert Pope and His American Dream Machines*, pp. 134-136; and Connecticut Historical Society collections.

Chapter Five: Moving on the Job Today: *Assembly Lines in Pennsylvania*
On-location visit to the Utz Potato Chip factory in Hanover, PA, November 10, 2005; Interview with Kris Shakely, occupational nurse.

(Cost of Model Ts and turnover rate at Ford Motor Co.) Robert Kanigel, *The One Best Way: Frederick Winslow Taylor and the Enigma of Efficiency,* Viking, 1997, pp. 495-498.

(doubling wages at Ford) Kanigel, *The One Best Way*, pp. 495-498.

Jeff Weinman, occupational therapist, Hanover Hospital, Hanover, PA; interview on location at plant on November 10, 2005.

(Quotation) Robert Kanigel, *The One Best Way,* Viking, 1997, p. 7.

(Shovel item) Kanigel, *The One Best Way*, pp. 2-3.

(Taylor at Packard) Kanigel, *The One Best Way*, p. 497.

(Taylor as a young man) Marta Braun, *Picturing Time: The Work of Etienne-Jules Marey,* University of Chicago Press, 1992, p. 337.

(Congressman) Robert Kanigel, *The One Best Way,* Viking, 1997, p. 3.

(Marey) Marta Braun, *Picturing Time,* University of Chicago Press, 1992. To see more of Marey's photos, visit www.marycollinswriter.net.

(Engineering as largest profession) Braun, *Picturing Time*, p. 335.

(Marey quotation) From Marey's book, *Animal Mechanism*, as quoted in Braun. Also used as background text in artwork in Dagognet, Francois, *Etienne Jules Marey: A Passion for the Trace*, translated from the French by Jeanine Herman, Zone Books, 1992.

(Invention of instruments) Braun, *Picturing Time,* p. xvii.

(Descriptions of workspace) Braun, *Picturing Time*; and Dagognet, *Etienne-Jules Marey*.

(Information on Janssen) Braun, *Picturing Time*; and Dagognet, *Etienne-Jules Marey*.

(70 paces item) Braun, *Picturing Time,* p. 206.

(Olympians) Braun, *Picturing Time*.

(Quotation about lecture) Braun, *Picturing Time*, p. 6-7.

On-location visit to Harley Davidson factory, November 10, 2005.

Chapter Six: Action and Stillness in Nature: *How Do Animals Achieve a Healthy Balance?*

(Sleep information) Carl Zimmer, "Down for the Count," *New York Times*, November 8, 2005, p. D1.

(Cheetah information): In-person interview, January 4, 2006, National Zoo, Washington DC, with John Gibbons, public affairs.

Anthony Hall-Martin, *Cats of Africa*, Smithsonian Institute Press, 1997.

Interview with John Gibbons and on-location personal observations; zoo visits December 30 and January 4.

(Zoo conservation efforts) interview with John Gibbons, public affairs.

(Specialists vs. opportunists) Desmond Morris, *The Human Zoo*, Kodansha International, originally published 1968 and reprinted in 1996, p. 184 (quotation) and p. 7 (impact on city dwellers).

(Hummingbirds) Robert Brown, *The World of Hummingbirds*, Gareth Stevens Publishing, 1991; Robert Burton, *The World of the Hummingbird*, Firefly Books, 2001; also personal observations at the cottage in NH.

(Sloth) Marco Ferrari, *Colors for Survival: Mimicry and Camouflage in Nature*, CIP, 1993; also Penelope Farrant, *Colour in Nature*, Blandford, 1997.

(Quick movers/slow movers' life span) Interview with John Gibbons, of the National

Zoo; Heinrich, *Winter World: The Ingenuity of Animal Survival,* Ecco, a division of Harper/Collins, 2003; movie at the Smithsonian Museum of Natural History's evolution exhibit [shrew ancestor]; Animal Planet, "Motion in the Extreme," TV special; Jozsef Stone, "Brief Lusty Life of the Mayfly," *National Geographic Magazine,* May, 2003; Hugh Colt, *Adaptive Coloration in Animals,* Methuen & Co., 1940; Attenborough, David, *Life of Birds,* Princeton University Press, 1998; "The Rise of Mammals Mothers of Us All," *National Geographic* magazine, April 2003; (insects and wings) Carl Zimmer, "A Pair of Wings Took Evolving Insects on a Nonstop Flight to Domination," *New York Times,* November 29, 2005, p. D3.

(Plants and movement) Bernd Heinrich, *The Trees in My Forest,* HarperCollins, 1997, pp. 89-104.

Charles Darwin and Francis Darwin, *The Power of Movement in Plants,* 1881.

(Bears and hibernation) Bernd Heinrich, *Winter World,* pp. 257-58; p. 260.

(Mouse study) Eric Blackstone, Mike Morrison, and Mark Rother, "Hibernating Mice May Someday Save Humans," *Science,* Vol. 308, Issue 5721, 518, 22 April 2005.

(Integrative exercise) Elizabeth Weil, "Fitness Can Be a Work in Progress," *New York Times,* October 27, 2005, p. C10.

Chapter Seven: Action and Stillness in Humans: *Can Americans Achieve a Healthy Balance?*

In-the-street visits in February, March, and August 2008.

(Information on Adams Morgan and Cleveland Park) DC Office of Latino Affairs, OLA.dc.gov; U.S. Census, QuickFacts.Census.gov/qfd/states/11000.html; DC government website for income averages, car drivers, etc, http://app.dchiz.dc.gov/info/pdf/Demographics.pdf

(Centers for Disease Control and Prevention [CDC] Quiz) CDC.gov/nccdphp/dnpa/physical/life/overcome/html

In-person interview with Matilde Palmer at the Family Place, 16th St., Washington, DC, March 16, 2008; in-person interviews with several women at the Family Place who would not give me their names.

In-person interviews with Rachel Winch and Harrison Taylor Godfrey in Cleveland Park on March 17, 2008; also their written journal entries.

(Prevention vs. medical) Thomas Farley and Deborah Cohen, *Prescription for a Healthy Nation: A New Approach to Improving Our Lives by Fixing Our Everyday World,* Beacon Press, 2005 (preventive history p. 18; quotations p. 238 and p. 154).

(General trends from 1960) J.D. Reed, "America Shapes Up," *Time,* November 2, 1981 (includes Terkel quotation); Dan Johnson, *The Futurist,* "Tracking Fitness: From Fashion Fad to Health Trend," May 1998; poll conducted by the American College of Sports Medicine as cited in an ABC news story: abclocal.go.com/Kabc/story?section=news/food_coach&id=6067401

(Yoga and Tai Chi) National Center for Complementary and Alternative Medicine: nccam.nih.gov/health/taichi/); general information from answers.com/topic/yoga?cat=health and the National Association of Tai Chi; Tai Chi Class Spring 2008, Unitarian Church, Albany Ave., Hartford, CT.

Chapter Eight: A Tour Through Sixty Years of Advice

(Centers for Disease Control and Prevention [CDC] Quiz) CDC.gov/nccdphp/dnpa/ physical/life/overcome/html

($32.4 billion figure) AHRQ.gov/ppip/activity.html

("Spontaneously active" observation) Health.gov/dietaryguidelines/dga2000/ document/aim.html

(25 percent increase in activity if more accessible places to be active) AHRQ.gov/ppip/ activity.html (and confirmed at ALR conference).

Juliet Schor, *The Overworked American: The Unexpected Decline of Leisure*, Basic Books, 1992. (sixteen hours of leisure a week, pg. 1; women with kids and jobs, hours worked, p. 21; quote about choice of hours, p. 128; low-energy leisure, p. 161).

(Creating bike lanes increases ridership) Active Living Research Center and National Center for Bicycling & Walking.

American Public Health Association, Washington, DC, Annual meeting, February 1, 2006, regarding National Public Health Week. Attended in person: APHA.org

(Statistics on membership and budget) APHA.org

(Information on marketing budget of AMA) *The Chicago Tribune*, May 23, 2006.

Keith Laughlin, director of Rails and Trails and attendee at APHA conference. In-person conversation, February 1, 2006.

(JFK program) Gina Kolata, *Ultimate Fitness: The Quest for Truth about Exercise and Health*, FSG, 2003 (p. 43 JFK; and 60 percent figure holding steady, p. 68).

(Anti-smoking material) Centers for Disease Control and Prevention, CDC.gov/nchs/ data (charts on smoking patterns in the United States. Official title of document *Health, United States 2005: Chartbook on Trends in the Health of Americans* (500 pages); also used Tobacoo.org/resources and *History of Cancer Prevention Studies*, Cancer.org

(Seatbelt use) "Buckling Up: Technologies to Increase Seat Belt Use," TRB Special Report 278, Transportation Research Board of the National Academies, Number 23, October 2003 and the National Highway Traffic Safety Administration website: PolicyAlmanac.org/economic/archive/seatbelts.shtml

(ALR) Active Living Research: ALR.com

Chapter Nine: Seeking Solutions in the Twenty-First Century

Personal observations in the airport at National Airport, Washington, DC, February 16, 2006.

Personal observations in San Diego and while flying, February 16, 2006.

Dr. James Sallis, program director of Active Living Research. Healthful choices quotation from *San Diego Tribune*, "Obesity: Is Personal Responsibility the Answer?" April 4, 2004, p. B-7; more academic work includes "Behavioral and Environmental Interventions to Promote Youth Physical Activity and Prevent Obesity," June 22, 2003, *Georgia Health Policy Center Report* (inconsistent suggestions on recommended daily activity requirement; various bullets on pages 3-4).

On location at the ALR Conference, February 17, 2006, Coronado Marriott Hotel. Personal observations of opening of conference, Dr. Terry Bazzare and Dr. James Sallis.

Matt Coogan, presenter, ALR Conference, February 17, 2006, "The Role of

Neighborhood Form and Personal Values in the Determination of Walk and Transit Mode," and lunch interview on February 17, 2006.

Dr. Susan Hardy, University of California, Davis, and presenter at ALR Conference, February 17, 2006, "Do Americans Want Walkable Communities?"

(New technologies for data collection) Dr. Weimo Zhu, Professor of Kinesiology at the University of Illinois at Urbana.

Toni Yancey, "Liftoff LA Style" leader, in-person observation, February 17, 2006, ALR conference.

(Blood pressure claim) Toni Yancey, ALR conference, February 17, 2006.

(Hurricane Katrina, numbers on devastation, LA mortality rates) Dr. Thomas Farley, Tulane University, ALR Conference Keynote Speaker, February 17, 2006.

(Bush pledge of $200 billion) film clip shown by Dr. Farley and figures for current amount pledged also Farley.

(PACE 2007) SPH.tulane.edu/PRC/pages/CoreResearch/html

Sharon Roerty, Executive Director, National Center for Bicycling & Walking, and in-person conversation at the ALR Conference evening of February 17, 2006.

(Louisville, KY, story) Roerty at ALR Conference and *The Courier-Journal,* May 31, 2005, and February 2005 articles, as well as Mayor Dave Armstrong's homepage and *Men's Health,* February 2006.

Sitting on plane with man reading *Making the Nation Safe* (personal observation, February 16, 2006 in flight to San Diego).

(Observations about people fleeing Twin Tower disaster) Sharon Roerty, interview February 17, 2006.

Chapter Ten: The Social Costs: *Trekking New York City for Answers*

(Statistics on number of children walking and biking to school) Active Living By Design newsletter.

On-location observations of MacArthur Elementary School, Alexandria, VA (2006); on-location observations of Gunston Middle School and Barrett Elementary School (2006), Arlington, VA, and Arlington County Government website, Arlington.K12.va.us

(Top ten most walkable cities) American Podiatric Medical Association. APMA.org

Sharon Roerty, in-person interview on location in Newark and Maplewood, NJ, and NYC; BikeWalk.org. On-location interviews and tour, April 30-May 1, 2006.

Jacobs, Jane, *The Death and Life of Great American Cities,* the Modern Library, 1993 edition (originally published in 1961); obituary, *New York Times,* April 26, 2006, by Douglas Martin; *New York Times* "Week In Review," "Outgrowing Jane Jacobs, by Nicolai Ouroussoff, April 30, 2006.

(SAFE-TEA-LU) Sharon Roerty and online at the National Center for Bicycling & Walking, "Safe Routes to School: Introduction," online newsletter.

(Area most densely packed in world) Ruth Limmer, *Six Heritage Tours of the Lower East Side,* New York University Press, 1997, p. 132.

(Number of Chinese in area and different languages) Patrick Radden Keefe, "The Snakehead," *The New Yorker,* April 24, 2006, p. 69.

(Mother at lunch) Constance Sullivan Collins Cain, Farmington, CT.

(Central Park facts) Roy Rosenzweig and Elizabeth Blackmar, *The Park and The People:*

A History of Central Park, Cornell University Press, 1992, p. 426 (quotation about park as piece of art; p. 26, information about keeping immigrants out of bars; p. 225; 1860 figures for foot traffic in park).

Also used for general information, Sara Cedar Miller, *Central Park: A Masterpiece,* Harry N. Abrams Inc., 2003; Bruce Bliven, *New York: A History,* W.W. Norton & Co. 1981; Peter Hamill, *Downtown: My Manhattan,* Little, Brown & Company; Peter Hamill, *Forever,* Thorndike Press, 2003.

(General sources for history) Jane Kay, *Asphalt Nation: How the Automobile Took Over America and How We Can Take It Back,* University of California Press, 1998.

James Kunstler, *The Geography of Nowhere: The Rise and Decline of America's Man-made Landscape,* Free Press, 1994.

"Creating Walkable Communities," prepared for the Mid-America Regional Council of Kansas City, MI by the Bicycle Federation of America, December 1998.

"Are We There Yet?" Assessing the Performance of State Departments of Transportation on Accommodating Bicycles and Pedestrians, Bill Wilkinson and Bob Chauncy, National Center for Bicycling & Walking, February 2003.

"Bringing Community to the City," *BusinessWeek,* by Pallavi Gogoi, February 2, 2006, about new urbanism taking hold and the Reston, VA-type development as most popular approach right now.

Lower East Side Tenement Museum, Tenement.org.

Chapter Eleven: A Spiritual Solution?

(Numbers on obesity and diabetes) Centers for Disease Control and Prevention, CDC. gov/od/oc/media/pressrel/fs040402/html; also "Latino Health Risks," small box of stats with no author in the *Washington Post,* January 17, 2006, p. F1.

(Four times as likely to be obese if don't feel safe) Amanda Gardner, *Healthday Reporter,* ABCNews, January 3, 2006. She cited Julie Lumeng, University of Michigan, who published a story about this in *Archives of Pediatrics and Adolescent Medicine.* Study also cited in the *Washington Post,* "Unsafe Neighborhoods, Overweight Kids," January 3, 2006.

(Hispanics at greater risk as walkers) AP story, December 2, 2005, "South's Hispanics far more likely to die walking," based on data from the Centers for Disease Control and Prevention, CDC.gov.

On-location observations on Route 1 in front of the Don Beyer Volvo car dealership, Fairfax, VA.

(African Americans and Hispanics as compared to Whites and Asians) Centers for Disease Control and Prevention, CDC.gov.

(Better access to food and Hispanic eating patterns) Malis M. Frenn, et. al, "Determinants of physical activity and low-fat diet among low income African Americans and Hispanics," *Public Health Nursing,* 2005, Mar-April 22 (2): 89-97.

Dr. Farley, keynote address, Active Living Research Conference, February 2006, San Diego, CA.

(Time issue) KC Heesch and LC Masse, "Lack of Time for Physical Activity: Perception or Reality for African American and Hispanic Women?" *Women Health* 2004 39 (3): 45-62.

(Comparing interests in African American vs. Caucasian girls) Marsha Dowda,

"Physical Activities and Sedentary Pursuits in African American and Caucasian Girls," *Research Quarterly for Exercise and Sport,* December 1, 2004.

(History of fitness ministries) Personal interview and on-location visit with Georgine Redmond, St. Anthony's Catholic Church, Falls Church, VA, May 21, 2006.

Marie R. Griffith, *Born Again Bodies: Flesh and Spirit in American Christianity,* University of California Press, 2004.

Ben Lerner, *Body by God: The Owner's Manual for Maximizing Living,* Nelson Books, 2003.

(Specific reference to distorted Fitness Ministry programs) Griffith, *Born Again Bodies.*

(Higher retention rates in exercise classes in churches) B.M. Kennedy and S. Paeratakul, et. al, "A pilot church-based weight loss program for African Americans adults using church members as health educators: a comparison of individual and group intervention," *Ethnic Dis.,* 2005 Summer; 15 (3) 373-8.

Jeannine Stein, "Body Work at Lord's Gym," the *Los Angeles Times,* Health Section, April 18, 2005, p. F1.

St. Paul's Journey, walking packet, Georgine Redmond.

Bible, Revised Standard Version.

Oxford English Dictionary, "Holy" and "Spirit"

On-location visit to Mount Olive Baptist Church, 1601 13 Road, S. Arlington, VA. LaVaeda Coulter, June 3, 2006.

Freddie, friend of LaVaeda's, on location at Mount Olive Church, June 3, 2006.

American Nursing Association, NursingWorld.org

Health Ministry Association: Hmassoc.org

INOVA Congregational Health Partnership (CIP) Peggy Steen.

Father Horace "Tuck" Grinnell, St. Anthony's Catholic Church. Phone interview, (June 2006).

Chapter Twelve: The Morality in Play

(Gardner's Multiple Intelligences Theory) pz.harvard.edu/pis/hg.htm and Howard Gardner, *Frames of Mind: The Theory of Multiple Intelligences,* April 2008 edition (25th anniversary edition).

(Hand-eye test) Charlottesville-Albemarle Technical School, Charlottesville, VA, 1989.

(Wright brothers story) From information I learned while writing *Airborne: A Photobiography of Wilbur and Orville Wright,* National Geographic Books, 2003, and while reporting for the Centennial of Flight edition of *Air & Space/ Smithsonian Magazine,* 2002.

(Laban/Bartenieff Institute) Limonline.org, and Karen Bradley, Washington, DC.

(Dog Whisperer story) Malcolm Gladwell, "What the Dog Saw: Cesar Millan and the movements of mastery," *The New Yorker,* May 22, 2006, pp. 52-53.

(Damasio and moral judgments) Antonio Damasio, *Descartes' Error: Emotion, Reason and the Human Brain,* Putnam Books, 1994, and quotations from an interview, Steven Johnson, "Antonio Damasio's Theory of Thinking Faster and Faster: Are the brain's emotional circuits hardwired for speed?" *Discover,* May 2004 pp. 45-49; Brain and Creativity Institute, University of Southern California, Los Angeles, CA.

(9/11 study) Richard Restak, *The New Brain: How the Modern Age Is Rewiring the Mind,* Rodale Press, 2003, pp. 77-79.

(Quotations from *Discover* interview) Steven Johnson, pp. 45-49.

($11,000 per year for health insurance) Julie Appleby, "Average Family Health Policy Nears $11,000," *USA Today*, Money Section, September 1, 2005.

(Fair to charge more for insurance if have unhealthy lifestyle and quotation) Robert Steinbrook, "Imposing Personal Responsibility for Health," *The New England Journal of Medicine*, August 25, 2006.

(Small company information) Vanessa Fuhrmans, "After Streak of Strong Profits, Health Insurers May See Decline," *Wall Street Journal*, July 31, 2006, p. A1.

(Poll of Americans) Fuhrmans, *Wall Street Journal*.

(West Virginia Study) Robert Steinbrook, "Imposing Personal Responsibility for Health," *The New England Journal of Medicine*, August 25, 2006.

(Ornish Study) Deutschman, Alan, "Why is it so darn hard to change our ways?" *Fast Company Magazine*, May 2005.

(Wii and stats on other games) John Gaudiosi, "How the Wii is creaming the competition," CNNMoney.com, April 25, 2007.

(*Wired Magazine*) Chris Anderson, "Welcome to the Broadband Home of the Future," *Wired*, Special Home Edition, 2004, pp. 7-16.

(My back surgeon) Dr. Jacobson, Washington Hospital Center, Washington, DC.

Chapter Thirteen: This Is Your Brain on Exercise

(Depression as a form of hibernation or brain lock) John Ratey and Eric Hagerman, *Spark: The Revolutionary New Science of Exercise and the Brain*, Little, Brown and Company, 2008, pp. 114-118 and 122-24; and specific quotation from psychiatrist Alexander Niculescu from an article in *Genome Biology*, 2005.

(Data on brain structure) Several sources: Ratey and Hagerman, *Spark*; and Arthur Bard and Mitchell Bard, *Understanding the Brain*, Pearson Educational Co., 2002, p. 75 (cerebellum) and p. 4 (energy supply).

(Embryo brain development) Lize Eliot, *What's Going on in There? How the Brain and Mind Develop in the First Five Years of Life*, Bantam Books, 1999.

(Direct Quotation) Eliot, *What's Going on in There?* p. 270.

(Chart of physical milestones) Eliot, *What's Going on in There?* p.262.

(Stories on brain exercises) Katie Hafner, "Exercise Your Brain or Else You'll . . . Uh . . ." *New York Times*, May 3, 2008, p. C 1.

(Miracle-Gro of the Mind and study of 5,000 elderly) John Ratey and Eric Hagerman, *Spark: The Revolutionary New Science of Exercise and the Brain*, Little, Brown and Company, 2008, p. 212.

(Lose 5 percent of brain volume) Ratey and Hagerman, *Spark*, p. 223.

(Only exercise can generate new neurons) Dr. Fred Gage, Salk Institute, in-person interview, La Jolla, CA, June 19, 2008.

(Description of how neurons and synapses develop) Lize Eliot, *What's Going on in There? How the Brain and Mind Develop in the First Five Years of Life*, Bantam Books, 1999, pp. 26-27.

(Cerebral Cortex triples in thickness in first year), Eliot, *What's Going on in There?* p. 27.

(Information about architecture of Salk and quotation about Picasso) Salk Institute brochure.

(50 percent of new cells die) Dr. Gage, Salk Institute.

(Basal ganglia, cerebellum, and brain stem) John Ratey and Eric Hagerman, *Spark: The Revolutionary New Science of Exercise and the Brain*, Little, Brown and Company, 2008, p. 42.
(Information on Dalai Lama) DalaiLama.com

Chapter Fourteen: Reclaiming Natural Grace in Natural Places: *Have You Had a Green Hour Today?*
(Circle of movement in kids) Richard Louv, *Last Child in the Woods: Saving Our Children from Nature-Deficit Disorder*, Algonquin Books of Chapel Hill, 2005, p. 123. He cited a study done by Sanford Gaster, "Urban Children's Access to Their Neighborhoods: Changes Over Three Generations," *Environment and Behavior*, January 1991, pp. 70-85.
Popham Beach, Maine, personal visit, July 10, 2006.
(Field trip observations) September 2006, Alexandria Country Day School, Alexandria, VA.
(Information about decibel levels) ReedCollege.com/ehs.health programs/noise and Quiet.org
Map, "Earth At Night," *National Geographic*, July 2004.
(Obesity vs. organized sports) Richard Louv, *Last Child in the Woods: Saving Our Children from Nature-Deficit Disorder*, Algonquin Books of Chapel Hill, 2005, p. 47.
(ADD treatment and time outside) Louv, *Last Child in the Woods*, p. 34.
(Depression/girls and view of green) Louv, *Last Child in the Woods*, p. 105.
(Cultural autism quotation) Louv, *Last Child in the Woods*, p. 64.
(Vocation as naturalist quote) Gary Paul Nabhan and Stephen Trimble, *The Geography of Childhood: Why Children Need Wild Places*, Beacon Press, 1994, p. 37.
(Hours outside as schoolboy) Nabhan and Trimble, *The Geography of Childhood*, p. 38.
(Quotation) Nabhan and Trimble, *The Geography of Childhood*, p. 94.
(Paul Bunyan), VisitBemidji.com
(Moving for video games) Crispin Boyer, "Video Game Central," *National Geographic for Kids*, August 2006, p. 15; Caroline Kettlewell, "Get A Move On," *Washington Post* Weekend Section, April 28, 2006, p. 30.
(Coyle interview) On-location in-person interview with Kevin Coyle, director of the Green Hour program at the National Wildlife Federation, Reston VA, June 29, 2006.
(Green Hour site) GreenHour.blogspot.com
(Carson) Rachel Carson, *A Sense of Wonder*, HarperCollins, first published in 1965 but used the 1998 reprint edition with photographs by Nick Kelsh, p. 17, p. 63, p. 66, p. 483.
(Carson liked going out at night) Linda Lear, *Rachel Carson: Witness for Nature*, Henry Holt and Co., 1997, p. 290.

Conclusion: Final Stop
(People who move live longer) Mayo Clinic study as reported in the *Washington Post*, "Simply Moving About May Help Extend Lives of Older People," July 18,

2006 (no byline) also see MayoClinic.com and Centers for Disease Control and Prevention, CDC.gov/aging.

(Kids who are active rather than tutored perform better on tests) Marvin Bynum, "Hand in Hand," *Athletic Business,* August 2005, an article that cites 200 plus studies that show ten minutes of activity before a task like reading or math problems is better than tutoring.

(WHO and 73 percent statistic) World Health Resolution WHA 57.17 also see WHO. int/dietphysicalactivity/en/ and update on 2004 report from the 59th World Healthy Assembly, "Implementation of Resolutions," May 11, 2006.

(Kaplan quotation) Marian Burros, "New Approach to Childhood Obesity Urged," *New York Times,* October 1, 2004, citing the National Academies' Institute of Medicine 2004 report on obesity, which was presented to Congress.

Sharon Roerty, Executive Director, Center for Bicycling and Walking, BikeWalk.org.

(Lunchroom material) Burkhard Bilger, "The Lunchroom Rebellion, *The New Yorker,* September 11, 2006.

(Statistics on Swedes) KidsRunning.com, which cited a study from *Medicine & Science in Sports & Exercise,* August 2003.

(Paid exercise breaks in Sweden) European Foundation for the Improvement of Living and Working Conditions.

(How these breaks more successful) Howard Tinsley, et. al, "Attributes of Leisure and Work Experiences," *Journal of Counseling Psychology,* 40 (1995) 447-55 also IUSB.edu/--journal/1998/paper17/html "Continuing Education During the Work Day," by Jamie Odem.

(USDL material) DOL.gov more specifically DOL.gov/dol/allcfr/Title_29/Part_ 785/29CFR785.18.htm

(Germans and gymnastics) Bill Sands, USOC.

(Eisenhower initiative) Fitness.gov/about_history.htm also UNM.edu.

(Overweight and unfit soldiers today) Army.mil/soldier/may95.

(Standards across various branches of military) StewSmith.com/linkpages/pft standards.htm.

D. H. Lawrence, poem, "Things Men Have Made."

Walt Whitman, *Complete Poetry and Selected Prose,* Houghton Mifflin, Riverside Editions, 1959, poems cited "The Body Electric" and "Song of Myself."

Suggested Steps for Building a Move Movement

We must all become more proactive about seeking *systemic changes* if we ever hope to finally crack that infamous 65 percent mark—the number of overweight or obese Americans who fail to engage in activity three to five times a week.

There's a lot of noise and information out there, but none of it will bring about substantial shifts among the general population without the political will and personal initiative on a scale with the anti-smoking campaigns.

To bring physical movement back into our everyday lives so that it flows like e-mail through our day:

- Pick targets such as improving the walkability of a town or the accessibility of public trails.
- Harness the power of established organizations to bring about change that's difficult for individuals to carry off on their own; for instance, employers could institute fifteen-minute paid movement breaks for desk workers. See the following "Resources" section for a list of organizations.
- Read the proposed Bill of Rights for the Move Movement on page 187.

To start your own private Move Movement:

- Begin with the Centers for Disease Control and Prevention (CDC) quiz at the end of this book on "Barriers to Being Active." In my case, time proved my biggest obstacle, so I needed to become more structured about adding movement to my daily life; not just organized exercise, but also casual activity, like walking for groceries, gardening, and working at a standup desk that encourages pacing. See the section on "Tips for Integrating Movement into Your Life," page 189.

- Track the activities of organizations, such as the Active Living Research Foundation and Rails to Trails, which stay on top of things like transportation bills that include requirements for bike trails. These organizations often provide state-by-state analysis and suggestions for getting involved politically and volunteering. See the following "Resources" section for a list of organizations and their websites.

Resources

ACCESS TO BETTER BIKING AND WALKING TRAILS
- National Center for Bicycling & Walking (BikeWalk.org)
- Rails to Trails Conservancy (RailsTrails.org)

ENCOURAGE MORE CHILDREN TO WALK TO SCHOOL
- National Center for Safe Routes to School (SafeRoutes/info.org)
- National PTA (PTA.org)

TRACK KEY TRENDS IN PHYSICAL ACTIVITY PATTERNS
- Active Living Research Foundation (ActiveLivingResearch.org)
- WE CAN (Ways to Enhance Children's Activity and Nutrition; sponsored by the U.S. Department of Health and Human Resources and the National Institutes of Health: NHLBI.nih.gov/health/public/heart/obesity/wecan)
- National Coalition for Promoting Physical Activity (NCPPA.org)
- Partnership for an Active Community Environment (PACE), Tulane University, Dr. Tom Farley: SPH.tulane.edu

PUSH FOR MORE WALKABLE COMMUNITIES
- Smart Growth Network (SmartGrowth.org/default.asp)
- Project for Public Spaces (PPS.org)

ENCOURAGE OUTDOOR ACTIVITIES FOR ALL, BUT ESPECIAL CHILDREN

◎   National Wildlife Federation (GreenHour.org)

The idea is to start thinking beyond the small changes you can make in your own life and start focusing on larger, long-term changes you can help create in your immediate world, from your neighborhood to your job. All of these organizations have advice for your general community, not just individuals. The National Wildlife Federation, for example, provides detailed suggestions on how the public schools in your district can better incorporate outdoor exercise and nature activities into recess and physical-education classes. You can pinpoint the problem and then lean on the organization's information to help you offer up a solution in your local district.

Our sedentary lifestyles evolved for many reasons, and it will take many different organizations and individuals to bring about real change—but it can and will happen.

Bill of Rights for the Move Movement

People with disabilities have made a lot of headway in the last fifty years when it comes to securing equal rights in the workplace, equal access to public spaces, and more. At this point, the physical life of the average American has become so truncated that they need a *Move Movement Bill of Rights* of their own, which addresses very similar problems.

- All Americans have a right to move on a regular basis at work in ways that are healthful and relieve mental and physical stress; the federal government should *require* all employers to allot two paid fifteen-minute movement breaks in a work day, especially for desk workers

- All Americans have a right to move in healthful ways in their own neighborhoods. Local and state governments should *require* all road repairs and new construction in heavily trafficked areas, like town centers, to incorporate pedestrian-friendly crosswalks, bicycle lanes, wider sidewalks, safe lighting, and greenery.

- All grammar and middle schools should be within walking distance of the children in the district. High Schools and other schools that cannot meet this criteria should be *required* to provide two fifteen-minute movement breaks during the school day that encourage free, noncompetitive, outdoor activity.

- All Americans have a right to live within walking distance of a safe public play space that does not require a permit to use.

- The federal government should create a Presidential Fitness Program for ALL American citizens, not just children K-8, which sets movement goals for every segment of a town's population. Government agencie at all levels—federal, state, and local—should be proactive about workin with people to help them meet these goals as a community.

◎ Sustaining some level of physical fitness is a civic obligation that the government, employers, schools, religious organizations, families, and individuals must work together to meet.

◎ To deny any of these rights is to undermine every citizen's right to happiness as set forth in the United States Constitution and risks leaving our citizenry depleted physically, mentally, and spiritually.

Tips for Integrating Movement
into Your Life

- There are many guidebooks out there on how much you need to move to stay healthy, but there's an easy way to sort through the noise. Remember that our hunter-gatherer ancestors moved about two to four miles a day (on about a third less calories than we take in). Use that as a healthy reference point for your activity patterns.

- No one likes to sit in sweaty clothes at work, but you should sweat everyday to clear toxins out of your system. Find out if your employer can install showers or team up with a local school or fitness center for "shower rights." You'll be more motivated to exercise rigorously on the way to work (walking or biking there, for example), if you can wash up.

- Allocate time and space for spontaneous free play in your life and your kids' lives. Most people are more active in unstructured settings. Don't let the organized sports leagues fool you; in general, they do not encourage enough exercise

- Employers need to break down the movement divide between work and leisure hours. Press for the right to paid movement breaks at work. Even fifteen minutes twice a day can result in a significant increase in focus and productivity.

- Desk work can be extremely hard on your dominate side. Right-handed people rarely train themselves to use a mouse with their left hand, for example. Work for more physical balance in front of your desk. Try a standup desk so you can sit and stand with ease. On a weekly basis, alternate which side you use your mouse.

- What's your movement/stillness ratio? Find out and improve on it. Do you sleep just six to seven hours a day and exercise only thirty minutes

twice a week? Healthier numbers: seven to eight hours of sleep a nig
and thirty minutes of exercise every day.

◎   Work with your neighbors to pressure your local grocery to offer more
fruits and vegetables. Insist that they cut back on the amount of shelf
space for soda, chips, and candy by 25 percent and replace it with
healthier choices.

◎   Make teenagers walk to school. Most live within easy walking or biking
distance, but take buses or cars. If they live too far away, demand that the
school integrate two fifteen-minute movement breaks (noncompetitive,
and preferably outside) into the school day.

◎   Every ten years, most municipalities resurface their roads. Insist that
your town include bicycling lanes and pedestrian-friendly routes along
streets near schools, including walk lights, wider sidewalks, and frequent
crossing points. Find out how the federal government's Safe-Routes-to-
Schools money in your state is being spent.

◎   For the overworked person who lives in a congested or unsafe area, a
local church can be a wonderful oasis, not just for spiritual and social
gatherings but for physical exercise. Use the Sunday quiet to begin
integrating physical activity back into your life.

◎   Watch people the next time you go to the grocery store and see how
they haphazardly move their carts, surprise each other because they never
"feel" anyone behind them, and generally move hesitantly through the
tightly crowded spaces. Where do you sit in the awkward dance? What's
your social movement IQ?

◎   Are you over fifty-five? Cut your chances of dementia in HALF by
engaging in physical activity every day. Many older people avoid places
with stairs and seek out flat living spaces, but studies show that as long
as your balance is sound, you're actually hurting your long-term health
and overall strength.

◎   Get outside. Move outside. Feel the sun and air on your face. Remember
an indoor life is a restricted, unhealthy life if lived to the urban extreme.

Centers for Disease Control and Prevention Quiz

Barriers to Being Active Quiz

What keeps you from being more active?

Directions: Listed below are reasons that people give to describe why they do not get as much physical activity as they think they should. Please read each statement and indicate how likely you are to say each of the following statements:

How likely are you to say?	Very likely	Somewhat likely	Somewhat unlikely	Very unlikely
1. My day is so busy now, I just don't think I can make the time to include physical activity in my regular schedule.	3	2	1	0
2. None of my family members or friends like to do anything active, so I don't have a chance to be physically active.	3	2	1	0
3. I'm just too tired after school/work to be active.	3	2	1	0
4. I've been thinking about becoming more physically active, but I just can't seem to get started.	3	2	1	0
5. Participating in physical activities can be risky.	3	2	1	0
6. I don't get enough exercise because I have never learned the skills for any one sport.	3	2	1	0
7. I don't have access to jogging trails, swimming pools, bike paths, etc.	3	2	1	0
8. Physical activity takes too much time away from other commitments—like work, family, etc.	3	2	1	0

9. I'm embarrassed about how I will look when I participate in physical activity with others.	3	2	1	0
10. I don't get enough sleep as it is. I just couldn't get up early or stay up late to be physically active.	3	2	1	0
11. It's easier for me to find excuses not to be physically active than to go out and do something.	3	2	1	0
12. I know of too many people who have hurt themselves by overdoing when they are physically active.	3	2	1	0
13. I really can't see learning a new sport.	3	2	1	0
14. It's just too expensive. You have to take a class or join a club or buy the right equipment.	3	2	1	0
15. My free times during the day are too short to include physical activity.	3	2	1	0
16. My usual social activities with family or friends do not include physical activity.	3	2	1	0
17. I'm too tired during the week and I need the weekend to catch up on my rest.	3	2	1	0
18. I want to be more physically active, but I just can't seem to make myself stick to anything.	3	2	1	0
19. I'm afraid I might injure myself.	3	2	1	0
20. I'm not good enough at any physical activity to make it fun.	3	2	1	0
21. If we had exercise facilities and showers at work/school, then I would be more likely to be physically active.	3	2	1	0

Follow these instructions to score yourself:

- ◉ Enter the circled number in the spaces provided, putting together the number for statement 1 on line 1, statement 2 on line 2, and so on.

- ◉ Add the three scores on each line. Your barriers to physical activity fall into one or more of seven categories: lack of time, social influences, lack of energy, lack of willpower, fear of injury, lack of skill, and lack of resources. A score of 5 or above in any category shows that this is an important barrier for you to overcome.

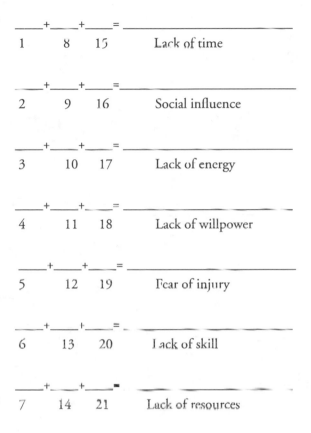

____+____+____= _____
1   8   15   Lack of time

____+____+____= _____
2   9   16   Social influence

____+____+____= _____
3   10   17   Lack of energy

____+____+____= _____
4   11   18   Lack of willpower

____+____+____= _____
5   12   19   Fear of injury

____+____+____= _____
6   13   20   Lack of skill

____+____+____= _____
7   14   21   Lack of resources

This Barriers to Being Active Quiz is used by permission from the SyberShop CD, North Carolina State University Cooperative Extension and A&T State University. Questionnaire is adapted from the "Barriers to Being Active" quiz in: U.S. Department of Health and Human Services, Public Health Service, Centers for Disease Control and Prevention, National Center for Chronic Disease Prevention and Health Promotion, Division of Nutrition and Physical Activity. *Promoting Physical Activity: A Guide for Community Action*. Champaign, IL: Human Kinetics, 1999 (available online at CDC.gov/nccdphp/dnpa/physical/life/barriers_quiz.pdf). For more information on the SyberShop CD, contact: North Carolina Cooperative Extension Service at 919.515.9142.

About the Author

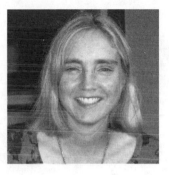

MARY COLLINS is a professor of creative writing at Central Connecticut State University and is the award-winning author of *The Essential Daughter: Changing Expectations for Girls at Home* (Praeger), *National Public Radio* (Seven Locks Press), and *Airborne: A Photobiography of Wilbur and Orville Wright* (National Geographic Books).

Ms. Collins has received numerous awards for her work, both as a professor and a writer, including the Best Essay of the Year Award from the American Society of Journalists and Authors (ASJA) and the Best Young Adult Book Award from ASJA as well. In addition, Ms. Collins has written many articles and books for a variety of clients, including *Smithsonian Magazine,* the *New York Times*, National Geographic Books, the Discovery Channel, the *Boston Globe*, Time-Life Books, McGraw-Hill, Pearson Publishing, and others.

Prior to teaching at Central Connecticut State University, Collins was an award-winning faculty member at Johns Hopkins University's graduate writing program in Washington, D.C. She remains actively involved in the professional writing community and is a sought-after panelist and speaker.